HEALING WATERS

The Powerful Health Benefits of Ionized H_2O

BEN JOHNSON, MD, DO, NMD

SQUAREONE
PUBLISHERS

The information and advice contained in this book are based upon the research and the personal and professional experiences of the author. They are not intended as a substitute for consulting with a health care professional. The publisher and author are not responsible for any adverse effects or consequences resulting from the use of any of the suggestions or procedures discussed in this book. All matters pertaining to your physical health should be supervised by a health care professional. It is a sign of wisdom, not cowardice, to seek a second or third opinion.

Cover Designer: Jeannie Tudor
Cover Photo: Getty Images, Inc.
Editor: Colleen Day
Typesetter: Gary A. Rosenberg

Square One Publishers
115 Herricks Road
Garden City Park, NY 11040
(877) 900-BOOK
www.squareonepublishers.com

Library of Congress Cataloging-in-Publication Data

Johnson, Ben, 1950 Nov. 11-
　Healing waters / Ben Johnson.
　　　p. cm.
　Includes bibliographical references and index.
　1. Acid-base imbalances—Diet therapy. 2. Water-electrolyte balance (Physiology) 3. Drinking water—Purification. 4. Antioxidants. I. Title.
　RM252.64 2011
　613.2'87—dc22

                              2011014676

ISBN 978-0-7570-0328-8

Printed in Canada

10　9　8　7　6　5　4　3　2　1

Contents

Introduction

Imagine if one of nature's most powerful healers was available to you twenty-four hours a day, seven days a week. Imagine if the answer to many of your most pressing health problems could be found in your own home. Though it may sound too good to be true, this is not a farfetched fantasy—it's a reality, and it's in your kitchen.

Water is the most abundant substance on earth, the primary source of life, and a liquid you consume in some form every day. It's in most of the foods you eat, it's the base for nearly every beverage you drink, and it's contained in every breath of air you inhale. So it's astonishing that so many medical conditions on the rise today stem from chronic dehydration—insufficient water intake over an extended period of time. From fatigue to premature aging, from asthma to inflammation, and from dry skin to diabetes, the body's need for more water often lies at the root of the problem. And although health professionals have touted the importance of proper hydration for several years, urging us to fit in our eight glasses daily, these problems remain. Why? Because when it comes to water's impact on your body, *quality* is just as important as *quantity*, especially for the prevention and treatment of disease. Meeting your daily water requirement is part of the battle, but the environmental toxins in tap water and our modern, highly acidic diet can counteract the numerous benefits offered by a glass of pure H_2O.

There's a way out of this dilemma. The solution is ionized water, which, for decades, has been used in other countries as a means of improving health. Superior to both distilled and filtered water, ionized water is H_2O that has undergone a mild—and safe—electrolyzing process that boosts its vitality, rids it of harmful acidifying chemicals, and makes it capable of transporting nutrients and oxygen all over your body quickly and effectively. Moreover, technological advances have made it possible for this scientific process to take place in your own home, which means that it can easily become part of your lifestyle and daily routine.

As a physician for more than thirty years, it has been my mission to spread the word about medical innovations that I have employed in my practice and found to work with my patients. Ionized water is one such innovation, and this book sets out to demystify the ionized water phenomenon, explaining the science behind the process of ionization as well as how it works to enhance practically every function your body carries out. Chapters 1 and 2 lay the groundwork for this investigation, beginning with a discussion of the health benefits of water in general and why the vast majority of Americans are suffering from the damaging effects of chronic dehydration. Chapter 2 is an informative guide to acid-alkaline balance, a major factor in maintaining good health. Acid-alkaline *imbalance* is connected to a wide variety of serious medical problems, and understanding this connection is one key to understanding the special power of ionized water.

Chapter 3 takes a closer look at ionized water and its distinctive characteristics. You'll learn about its chemical makeup and how it came to be used for medicinal purposes. In this chapter you will also discover how electrolysis improves the quality of drinking water more than distillation or filtration. Chapter 4 introduces the two key properties of ionized drinking water—high pH and antioxidant strength. The information in this chapter will help you better understand the numerous health benefits offered by alkaline ionized water, which are covered in Chapter 5 and include allergies, diabetes, and premature aging. Chapter 6 then turns to acidic ionized water and its practical uses, such as skin care and oral hygiene.

The final two chapters of this book are geared towards you, the reader, and give some guidelines for not only making ionized water a part of your everyday life, but also maximizing its benefits. Chapter 7 provides dietary recommendations and food-combining tips for achieving acid-alkaline balance. Foods and beverages have been categorized according to their acidifying or alkalizing effects, which will help you make dietary choices that reinforce ionized water's healing function. Chapter 8 is a helpful guide to buying and using a water ionizer, an investment that will surely change the way you live for the better. You can also consult the "Resources" section at the end of the book to find ionizer manufacturers and distributors located in the United States.

Simply put, ionized water is nature's water. Reading this book is the first step towards total rejuvenation of your body and overall health. If you want to enrich the quality of your health and life naturally, safely, easily, and in the comforts of your own home, then read on.

1

Water and Your Health

It's no secret that drinking water is essential for good health. The human body is approximately 65 percent water, so when you are deprived of it, you simply cannot survive. Without water, every cell, tissue, and organ in your body would go without oxygen and nutrients. Hormone and brain chemical levels would drop significantly, impairing neurological and endocrine function. You would be in a constant state of fatigue. In short, it would be impossible for your body to achieve, much less maintain, homeostasis—internal stability and balance.

Despite these facts, many people do not meet their daily water requirements and, therefore, live with symptoms of a condition they don't even know they have. Chronic dehydration, a problem largely connected to poor diet and eating habits, is often an unknown cause of disease. The prevalence of chronic dehydration is one of the main reasons why drinking ionized water is an effective way to improve your health. But before discussing how ionized water can alleviate dehydration, a general overview of water and its benefits may be useful. In the following pages, you'll find out how essential water is to your health, including the many roles it plays in the body. Additionally, this chapter provides some basic facts about chronic dehydration and explains how the condition is linked to another national health crisis—obesity.

WATER: A BIOLOGICAL NECESSITY

Water is the main substance and source of life, possessing a number of properties that make it integral to your body's function and performance. In addition to acting as a natural cleanser, water is the body's primary solvent, dissolving vital substances so that your cells can absorb them. In fact, the nutrients you take in from food sources do not have any inherent energy value until they are dissolved in water, which is an essential part of the digestive process. Nutrients are metabolized and assimilated only after they are broken down into smaller particles—a function facilitated by water. This is also true for oxygen, which is transported through the bloodstream and distributed to your cells by water. In other words, the oxygenation and nutritional nourishment of the body is entirely dependent on the presence of H_2O.

Water is also responsible for powering your cells, literally generating electrical and magnetic energy inside each and every one of your trillions of cells' *mitochondria,* or energy factories. Furthermore, water serves as the cells' primary bonding agent, enabling them to maintain their proper structure. This function is crucial for cellular maintenance, since a loss of structural integrity can eventually lead to disease. For instance, damaged DNA—which is contained in the nucleus of nearly every cell in your body—can cause abnormal cell behavior. As health experts have discovered, cellular abnormalities are a known cause of cancer and other serious medical conditions. But with adequate water, your cells are able to rid themselves of harmful toxins and strengthen the body's ability to ward off disease.

Water enables proper physiological function in more general ways as well, aiding in the following bodily processes:

- Elimination of waste products (via urination)

- Immune function

- Joint lubrication

- Liver and kidney function

- Lymphatic function

- Muscle function

- Production of hormones and neurotransmitters

- Regulation of body temperature (via perspiration)

- Respiration

- Skin maintenance

Considering water's central role in the body, it's hardly surprising that insufficient amounts of this liquid can take its toll on your internal balance. However, the extent to which inadequate water intake can impair the body was not known until relatively recently. Early research on chronic dehydration, as well as water's medicinal uses, is discussed in the next section.

THE DISCOVERY OF CHRONIC DEHYDRATION

The condition now known as chronic dehydration was first discovered in an Iranian prison in 1979, where Dr. Fereydoon Batmanghelidj, who had received his medical training at London University's St. Mary's Hospital Medical School, was detained as a political prisoner. He began to study the healing effects of water after another inmate was brought to his cell with pain caused by a severe peptic ulcer. Because he did not have any medicine at his disposal, Dr. Batmanghelidj instructed the man to drink two glasses of water every three hours to alleviate the pain. By doing so, the prisoner was pain-free for the four months that remained of his sentence. This breakthrough surprised and excited the doctor, who went on to treat more than 3,000 cases of peptic ulcer using this method during the three years he spent in prison. In fact, Dr. Batmanghelidj overstayed his sentence for the sole purpose of conducting more research, and by the time he left in 1982, his findings had been published in the *Journal of Clinical Gastroenterology* and *The New York Times.*

By studying his fellow prisoners, Dr. Batmanghelidj concluded not only that many serious health problems are caused by a water deficit, but also that such problems can be remedied simply by drinking more water. In the years that followed his release from prison, Dr. Batmanghelidj went on to discover the potency of water in treating a number of conditions, including:

- Addictive urges related to alcohol, caffeine, and various drugs
- Anxiety, depression, and stress
- Arthritis
- Asthma
- Attention-deficit disorders in both adults and children
- Back, joint, and muscle pain
- Blood clots
- Constipation and diarrhea
- Edema
- Fatigue
- Gastrointestinal problems
- Glaucoma
- Heart disease
- High blood pressure
- Hot flashes
- Impotence and loss of libido
- Insomnia and other sleep disorders
- Kidney stones
- Lupus
- Memory problems
- Morning sickness during pregnancy

- Premenstrual syndrome (PMS)

- Respiratory and sinus problems

- Urinary tract infections

The connection between water deprivation and disease led Dr. Batmanghelidj to conclude that many people suffer from *chronic dehydration,* or a state in which the body, denied adequate amounts of water for a prolonged period, cannot carry out activities efficiently, if at all.

To get an idea of what happens to the cells and tissues of your body when dehydration sets in, consider a piece of fruit set out on a countertop. If it is not eaten, before long, it will begin to dry out, shriveling up both inside and out as its water supply is depleted. Something similar happens to the cells and tissues in your body when you are dehydrated: They literally begin to wrinkle, losing their structural integrity and ability to function properly. The body, in turn, is unable to maintain homeostasis, which increases its susceptibility to a number of health problems.

As Dr. Batmanghelidj recognized, water deficits produce several symptoms that are seemingly unrelated to a low water supply. In addition to chronic pain, symptoms that also may arise include acne, digestive problems, dry skin and eyes, fatigue, headaches, irritability, muscle soreness, and sinus pressure, among others. The best way to prevent such symptoms is to drink water throughout the day, but dehydration may still occur depending on certain factors such as diet, climate, illness, and level of physical activity. See the inset on page 10 for information about determining whether you are sufficiently hydrated.

WHY ARE WE CHRONICALLY DEHYDRATED?

Chronic dehydration can develop for a number of reasons, but the primary and most obvious of these is poor eating and drinking habits. A sufficient amount of water in your body is dependent on consistent hydration throughout the day, as well as eating behav-

Are You Chronically Dehydrated?

"How do I know if I'm dehydrated?" is a question I'm constantly asked by patients. Most people mistakenly assume they only need to pay attention to signs such as dry mouth and extreme thirst to determine whether their body is water deprived. However, as Dr. Batmangheldij's studies repeatedly suggest, a dry mouth is actually the *last* outward sign of chronic dehydration. This is because feelings of thirst develop long after your body's water supply has fallen below the level needed for optimal functioning.

Rather than waiting until you feel thirsty, gauge your body's water needs by monitoring your urine, which is probably the easiest and most accurate way to know if you need to drink more water. A well-hydrated body produces urine that is clear; a slightly to moderately dehydrated body produces bright yellow urine; and finally, a body that is chronically dehydrated produces urine that appears orange or dark-colored. Sometimes the use of certain vitamins or other nutritional supplements can change the color of your urine. But if you do not take supplements and your urine appears dark in color, you should immediately increase your water intake and consult a health practitioner as a precaution.

iors that promote a healthy water level. Let's examine each of these factors more closely.

Inadequate Hydration

Every day, your body loses water naturally through the course of its activities. The average adult loses about three to four quarts of water per day due to breathing (exhalation), perspiration, urination, and the elimination of bodily wastes in the form of feces. Breathing alone accounts for approximately one to two quarts of this water loss. Moreover, there are circumstances that can affect the amount the body loses. Exercise, high altitudes, and warm climates can all increase your daily water loss. Illness may also cause a decrease in water level, especially if fever or diarrhea occurs. And this is not to mention the times when you may pour out a glass of tap or bottled water because its color, taste, or smell is off-putting.

Although you are protecting your body from toxic chemicals, you still are not hydrating your system.

Chronic dehydration sets in because people neglect to compensate for this natural water loss by keeping themselves hydrated throughout the day. Instead, most drink water or some other beverage only when they begin to experience acute thirst. This is a big mistake, according to Dr. Batmanghelidj, who found that thirst signals are felt several hours *after* the body initially becomes dehydrated. During this time, a variety of problems can arise, producing symptoms such as dry skin, fatigue, joint soreness, and muscle aches.

Eating Habits

It may come as a surprise that your eating habits can have a profound effect on the amount of water in your body. But think about how you respond to a drop in energy, which is one of the first and most noticeable signs that your water supply needs to be replenished. Do you try to eliminate this energy deficit with a glass of water, or do you reach for a snack, soft drink, or other unhealthy substitute? If you're like most people, your answer is probably the latter—and both cultural and physiological factors are to blame.

When your energy plummets, a chain reaction is set off in your body. The brain releases histamine, a chemical that stimulates hunger by causing sensations in the mouth and stomach. The problem is that this chain reaction that results in hunger is also initiated when you are thirsty, and your brain cannot distinguish between these two needs. In other words, if you are not well-attuned to your physical needs, you may easily confuse thirst with hunger, and then immediately attempt to boost your energy with food instead of water. This confusion is compounded by the fact that a drop in energy usually produces sugar cravings, so the foods instantly turned to are ones high in carbohydrates and sugar. A vicious cycle of low energy, unnecessary eating, and continued water deprivation ensues, and the ultimate consequence is chronic dehydration— not to mention weight gain.

CHRONIC DEHYDRATION AND OBESITY

Considering that how and what you eat can contribute to chronic dehydration, it makes sense that many people who are chronically dehydrated are also overweight or obese. As explained in the previous section, fatigue is one of the most common symptoms of insufficient water consumption. Having low energy not only increases your tendency to overeat, but also makes you less inclined to engage in physical activity. In addition, studies have shown that because drinking water influences your metabolism, an inadequate supply reduces the body's ability to burn fat. The likely result is excess fat storage, particularly on the waist, thighs, and buttocks. Water retention—which results when the body senses its water supply is running low—can also add extra pounds and produce symptoms typically associated with obesity, such as bloating, sagging skin, and edema, a disorder marked by swollen wrists and ankles.

Fortunately, both chronic dehydration and obesity are reversible conditions. German scientists at the Franz Volhard Clinical Research Center in Berlin found that people could lose weight by increasing their water intake by 1.5 liters a day—approximately 51 ounces. This amount, they estimated, can help burn an additional 17,400 calories—the equivalent of five pounds—in a single year. Simply put, by rehydrating the body, weight can be controlled and kept at a healthy level, as water both provides energy and curbs the appetite. Dr. Batmanghelidj himself discovered that overweight people who consumed two 8-ounce glasses of water before or after each meal were better able to distinguish between thirst and hunger, and they began to eat less, both in quantity and frequency. These findings suggest that drinking enough water goes a long way in fighting what many consider to be the most serious health issue facing our population today.

MEETING YOUR DAILY WATER REQUIREMENT

The question still remains: How can you ensure that you're satisfying your body's water needs every day? As a general rule, you should aim to drink at least one-half of an ounce of water per pound of body weight. This means that if you weigh 130 pounds, you should drink a minimum of 65 ounces of water daily, which works out to slightly more than eight 8-ounce glasses of water. The table below lists daily water requirements according to weight. However, keep in mind that these recommendations do not account for factors such as physical activity, climate, or illness, all of which affect how much water you should drink.

RECOMMENDED WATER INTAKE	
Body Weight (lbs.)	Daily Water Requirement (oz.)
100–120	50–60
121–140	60–70
141–160	70–80
161–180	80–90
181–200	90–100
201–220	100–110
Greater than 221	Greater than 110

By planning out your glasses of water and sticking to a regular schedule, meeting your daily requirement is very feasible. However, it's equally important to pay attention to your body's signals and drink whenever you're thirsty. By being attuned to your level of thirst, as well as monitoring the color of your urine (see inset on page 10), you will be in a better position to judge whether or not you're adequately hydrated. Here are some other suggestions for maintaining a proper amount of H_2O in your body:

- Avoid soda, which is full of artificial additives and highly dehydrating. The same goes for commercial non-herbal teas like green, black, and oolong tea. Instead, try making your own tea by adding fruits like lemons, oranges, or apples to boiling water.

- Beware of bottled water, since the plastic contains unhealthy chemicals that can easily leach into the water and compromise its nutritional value.

- Get in the habit of drinking a glass of water or two before every meal. Doing so supports digestion and reduces hunger pangs, which will promote healthier eating habits.

- Increase your consumption of water-rich foods. Fruits and vegetables such as apples, broccoli, tomatoes, and watermelon have high water content, as do eggs and yogurt.

- Limit your consumption of coffee and alcoholic beverages as much as possible, as they are both very dehydrating. Rather than start your morning with a caffeine fix, drink a large glass of water before breakfast—it will both energize you and fill you up.

- Take regular "water breaks" throughout the day, or carry a glass or stainless steel water bottle with you to refill as needed.

Additionally, Dr. Batmanghelidj recommended that people consume one-quarter teaspoon of salt (sea or Celtic) per 32 ounces of water. This ensures an adequate mineral supply is maintained. By following these useful tips and modifying water intake when necessary (due to factors such as exercise, for example), you will begin to notice a positive difference in how you feel.

CONCLUSION

Although drinking water is essential to your health, it has become more and more difficult to ensure that the water you're drinking is actually good for you. As you probably already know, much of our drinking water contains contaminants that make H_2O more harmful than healing. Drinking water filled with acidifying toxins not only complicates the problem of chronic dehydration, but also compounds the problem of acid-alkaline imbalance—which is already common due to poor eating and lifestyle habits. Ionized water is the solution to both of these health issues, and you will find out why in Chapter 3. But first, you should understand the importance of acid-alkaline balance to your overall health, and how the quality of your drinking water can dramatically affect it.

2

The Problem of Acid-Alkaline Imbalance

One of the most groundbreaking nutritional discoveries in recent years is the fact that every food you eat has a significant effect on your internal balance. Some foods and beverages have an acidifying effect upon being digested by the body, while others are alkalizing and neutralize potentially harmful acids. Due to our biology and genetics, all human beings must achieve a state of acid-alkaline balance in order to maintain good health. Unfortunately, biological necessity is often incompatible with modern dietary habits, which tend to keep our bodies in a state of mild *acidosis*, or slight over-acidity. As I mentioned in the previous chapter, drinking water that is acidifying—and much of our tap water is—can worsen acidosis, leading to a number of serious diseases. In order to understand why ionized water is the solution to this problem, you should first be familiar with acid-alkaline balance and how crucial it is to your well-being.

WHAT IS ACID-ALKALINE BALANCE?

Simply put, *acid-alkaline balance* refers to the balance between the amount of *acids* and *alkalis* (non-acids) in your body tissues and fluids—mainly blood, saliva, and urine. The ratio of acids to non-acids is determined by measuring *pH*, a term literally meaning "potential for hydrogen," which is used to represent the relative concentration of hydrogen ions, simple *protons* (positively charged particles), in blood, urine, and saliva. First defined by Danish biochemist Søren Peter Lauritz Sørenson in 1909, pH is used to measure the acidic, alkaline, or neutral properties of various solutions and compounds as well as the body's fluids and tissues.

pH is measured on a scale of 0 to 14. A measurement of 7 is neutral, being neither acidic nor alkaline. Measurements lower than 7 are considered acidic, while measurements higher than 7 are considered alkaline. As the number of hydrogen ions in a substance increases, so does the substance's level of acidity. To put it another way, acids give off hydrogen ions, and alkalis (or bases) accept hydrogen ions. For optimal health, your body's blood chemistry needs to be slightly alkaline, having a pH reading of 7.38 to 7.42. When your pH reading moves too far below or above this number for an extended period of time, disease or illness is usually the result.

Doctors have recognized the link between pH balance and disease since the early twentieth century, and today they know more about the detrimental consequences of acid-alkaline imbalance. Although there are rare cases of over-alkalinity (termed *alkalosis*), acidosis is the far more common problem, especially in the United States. Acidosis, or chronic over-acidity, results when the acids of the various substances you take in build up to a point where your body is no longer able to successfully neutralize or eliminate them. Over-acidity also creates an oxygen-deprived blood environment and supports the growth of unhealthy microorganisms in the bloodstream, including bacteria, fungi, mold, yeasts (such as *Candida*), and viruses. Other serious health conditions associated with acid-alkaline imbalance are discussed beginning on page 17.

ACID-ALKALINE BALANCE AND WATER

Today, much of the drinking water available to us is acidifying due to both external factors (such as pollution) and water's chemical makeup, which includes hydrogen ions. Chapter 3 explains the science behind hydrogen ions and the process of ionization. For now, you should understand some basic facts about hydrogen ions in water and their relationship to your body's pH level.

Along with oxygen, hydrogen is the main component of water, which is made clear by its chemical representation: H_2O. Hydrogen ions are formed as part of water's chemical reaction, and the higher the concentration of hydrogen ions, the more acidic the water. The concentration of hydrogen ions is minuscule in pure water, and although there is a slightly higher concentration in tap water, its overall pH reading is not significantly affected. Still, because hydrogen ions are inherently unstable and very reactive, they "hide" in your body's water, waiting to attach themselves to other molecules. This results in reactions between acids (which give off hydrogen ions) and alkalis (which accept hydrogen ions), thus altering your pH balance.

Acidic toxins, which are contained in tap water due to chemical treatments and environmental pollution, increase the concentration of hydrogen ions in the water you drink regularly. Most drinking water has a high chloride content, making it even more acidic. In addition, scientists have recently discovered the presence of pharmaceutical drugs—also very acidic—in much of the nation's water supply. The true extent of the internal harm caused by these chemicals remains to be seen, but it's been determined that their high concentration of hydrogen ions affects the pH level of water, in turn upsetting acid-alkaline balance when consumed.

THE CONSEQUENCES OF ACID-ALKALINE IMBALANCE

Extreme, life-threatening cases of acid-alkaline imbalance are relatively rare, but even slight acidosis can harm the body and profoundly affect its overall function and energy level. This section highlights some major and increasingly common health problems that stem from over-acidity in the body.

Accelerated Aging

Accelerated aging, also known as *premature aging,* is the direct result of weakened cellular structure, which occurs when cells are continually exposed to an overly acidic environment. Just as when the body is dehydrated, over-acidity causes the cell walls to shrivel, so that, when viewed under a microscope, the cells appear bent and misshapen. This loss of structural integrity affects the cells' ability to function properly, "communicate" with other cells, and manufacture the proteins essential for repair. In particular, acidosis impedes the production of *heat shock protein*, which facilitates the regenerative process. An inadequate amount of heat shock protein can trigger premature cell death, potentially resulting in impaired organ systems as well as shortages of substances vital for healthy, wrinkle-free skin, such as collagen and elastin.

Over-acidity also negatively affects brain function, which, of course, is associated with the aging process. Acidosis inhibits the proper function of *neurons*, nerve cells that help initiate and conduct brain impulses. When neurons lose the ability to work efficiently, mental acuity decreases, producing side effects such as confusion, forgetfulness, and "brain fog"—a state characterized by lack of clarity and focus. Moreover, though it has yet to be verified by science, there's reason to believe that there is a strong connection between chronic acidosis and Alzheimer's. A study conducted in 2006, for example, found a correlation between a gene influential in the development of Alzheimer's and insufficient oxygen levels in the body—a condition that is linked to over-acidity. (See page 44 for more about this Alzheimer's study.)

Demineralization

Your body draws upon its alkaline mineral stores in order to buffer or neutralize excess acids in your fluids and tissues. While the occasional withdrawal of these minerals is not likely to pose a problem, chronic acidosis means a substantial loss of minerals—including calcium, potassium, and magnesium—that are crucial to your well-being. Since these minerals are stored in all body tissues, their depletion can greatly affect your organ function. Less serious side effects include brittle nails, dry and cracked skin, sensitive gums, and thinning hair. But it's your bones and teeth that are especially affected by demineralization.

Dr. Susan Brown, a world-renowned expert in osteoporosis, has pointed out that demineralization is virtually nonexistent in cultures where whole foods, which promote acid-alkaline balance, are regularly eaten. In her book, *Better Bones, Better Body*, Dr. Brown states, "In our society, we consume a very imbalanced diet high in acid-forming foods. This imbalanced diet pushes us towards an acid state...[E]xcessive and prolonged acidity can drain bones of calcium reserves and lead to bone thinning." As this thinning process occurs, bones lose their flexibility, increasing the risk of osteoporosis and age-related fractures. Spinal discs may deteriorate, thereby increasing the potential for chronic back pain and sciatica. Rheumatism, a condition caused by inflamed joints, can also develop.

Demineralization can result in dental problems as well, because the loss of calcium makes teeth more brittle and prone to chipping. Teeth may also develop sensitivities to hot and cold foods, and become more susceptible to cavities. Tooth decay, common among children today, is almost always caused by a steady diet of foods like sugary cereal, soda, and fast-food meals, which, of course, are acid-forming.

Fatigue

Fatigue is one of the most frequently experienced symptoms of acid-alkaline imbalance. The reason is simple: Acidosis creates an internal environment that is not conducive to optimal energy production. This is because over-acidity diminishes the body's supply of oxygen, one of the main sources of energy. A depleted oxygen level prevents normal cellular function, leading to fatigue.

Further problems arise when the body's internal environment is *anaerobic* (lacking oxygen) for a significant period of time. Toxins and harmful microorganisms flourish and proliferate when cells, deprived of oxygen, cannot function properly. These toxins interfere with the body's ability to absorb and utilize nutrients such as vitamins, minerals, and amino acids, in turn making hormone and enzyme production more difficult. Cellular repair, organ activity, and blood-sugar maintenance are all affected when the body cannot manufacture these biochemicals, resulting in greater fatigue and less physical endurance. Microorganisms such as yeasts and fungi can also disturb electrolyte balance, reducing the normal flow of energy in the body. If left unchecked, this can lead to chronic fatigue syndrome (CFS), which explains why people who suffer from CFS invariably also suffer from acidosis. In my experience with patients, it is the acidosis that came first.

Impaired Enzyme Activity

Enzymes are chemical substances that literally make life possible. They are necessary for every process that your body carries out, including digestion, immune function, reproduction, respiration, and overall organ function. Enzymes are also required for cerebral functions such as movement, speech, and thought, and proper levels are needed in order for hormones, vitamins, and minerals to perform their various tasks.

Your body produces thousands of different types of enzymes, and each acts as a catalyst for a particular biochemical reaction. However, enzymes can initiate these chain reactions only within a specific pH level. When blood pH is too acidic, enzyme function is disrupted or sharply declines, allowing illness to take hold. Although mild at first, the illness can quickly progress if measures are not taken to restore proper acid-alkaline balance. When enzyme function completely shuts down due to unhealthy pH levels, the situation becomes life-threatening.

To safeguard against such damaging effects, many health practitioners recommend digestive and metabolic enzyme supplements. Though supplementation treats the enzyme dysfunction, correcting the problem entirely depends on restoring acid-alkaline balance through dietary and lifestyle modifications.

Inflammation and Organ Damage

The excess acids that build up due to chronic acidosis can harm the organs and tissues with which they come into contact, creating inflammatory conditions. Although over-acidity can cause inflammation anywhere in the body, the kidneys and skin, the organs through which acids are eliminated, are particularly affected. When the amount of acid is too great for the skin and kidneys to dispose of easily, a number of problems may arise. Skin blotching, eczema, hives, and itching can occur as a direct result of acidic sweat passing through the sweat glands. When exiting the body via the kidneys, excess acid may inflame the urinary tract, causing a painful burning sensation during urination. Very often, this leads to urinary tract infections and cystitis—inflammation of the bladder.

Compounding this problem is the fact that acid buildup also impairs immune function. White blood cells, which are responsible for targeting and destroying microbial invaders, are reduced in quantity as well as quality when your body is overly acidic. A weakened internal environment allows various tissues to become infected by the microorganisms that penetrate damaged cells, leading to more serious infections and inflammatory conditions.

Growth of Harmful Microorganisms

When the pH of the blood remains consistently below 7.38, the bloodstream becomes a breeding ground for harmful microorganisms, much like a stagnant swamp. This happens because acidosis reduces the available oxygen supply in the bloodstream, and many microorganisms thrive in the absence of optimum oxygen levels.

In 1931, the German scientist Dr. Otto Heinrich Warburg (1883–1970) was awarded the Nobel Prize in Medicine for his discovery that cancer cells flourish in low-oxygen environments. When the oxygen supply in the bloodstream is diminished, cells revert to what Warburg called a "primitive" state. In other words, the cells begin to derive their energy from glucose rather than oxygen. The process that makes glucose available to cells is fermentation, which produces a substance known as lactic acid. This acid further diminishes the body's oxygen and increases its level of acidity. This oxygen-deficient state causes cells to devolve and, in some cases, become cancerous. (See page 45 for more about the relationship between cancer and oxygen levels.)

A low-oxygen environment is also responsible for the growth and spread of microorganisms such as bacteria, fungi, molds, yeasts (including *Candida albicans*), and viruses in the body, all of which ferment glucose. In addition, they reproduce by using the fat and proteins needed for cellular regeneration and other vital functions. In this way, the microorganisms are able to spread all over the body, targeting weak areas, breaking down tissues, and interfering with essential bodily processes.

The most serious health problem posed by microorganisms, though, is not the microorganisms themselves, but the waste products they produce during their life cycle. These excretions are also acidic, and they further pollute your body and invade your cells as they are released into the bloodstream. As the microorganisms spread, disease develops and worsens over time.

DETERMINING YOUR PH

Now that you know how important acid-alkaline balance is to your health, you probably want to learn how to determine if your pH level is within a healthy range. Luckily, tests for measuring pH are readily available and can be either self-administered or performed by a physician. Two common testing procedures are explained in detail below.

Venous Plasma pH Test

The venous plasma pH test provides an accurate reading of your blood pH, so it can literally be life-saving. However, this test can be performed only by a doctor or health practitioner because it requires a blood sample, which is then sent to a licensed laboratory for a thorough analysis. If you decide to have this test, you should request that the measurement be made to the nearest one-hundredth of a point. A reading of 7.36 or 7.25, for example, is much more precise than 7.3 or 7.2.

Because of how important blood pH levels are to your overall health, I recommend that you make the venous plasma pH test part of your annual physical check-up. You should request the test when you schedule your appointment, as it is not commonly administered. The additional cost is nominal—less than one hundred dollars, depending on the lab used or recommended by your doctor—and the information it provides is invaluable.

The pH Strip Test

If you would rather self-administer a test at home, you can buy pH strips from your local drugstore. They may also be available at a health food store in your area. pH strips are made of litmus paper, which changes color when it comes into contact with alkaline or acidic substances. A color chart is included with the strips to help you gauge your pH as accurately as possible. But in general, testing with pH strips is less precise than a blood test.

Unlike the venous plasma test, pH strips require only a saliva or urine sample. Since the pH of saliva can have a wide variance, I recommend using urine. The test is simple. Take a pH strip and moisten it with your urine as you urinate—a quick dip into your urine stream is all that is necessary. As the acid content of your urine reacts with the pH strip, the strip will change color. Usually, shades of red and orange will indicate acidity, while blue is a sign of alkalinity. However, tests may vary, so you should match the color of the strip to the accompanying chart. In addition, pay attention to the shade of the color of the strip, as this will tell you how extreme or mild your pH reading is. A light shade of red, for instance, means that your body is slightly over-acidic, while a deeper shade is an indication of a more serious imbalance.

Since urine pH values can change during the day in reaction to the foods you eat, the best time to measure urine pH is in the morning soon after you've awakened and before you eat breakfast. And because a urine pH test does not give an exact reading of your body's internal acid-alkaline balance, I suggest performing this test five mornings in a row to get a better idea of your pH. If your reading is consistently within the range of 7.0 to 7.5, your body is in a fairly healthy state of acid-alkaline balance.

CONCLUSION

Acid-alkaline balance is one of the keys to optimal health. An imbalanced state, when sustained for an extended period of time, can lead to chronic degenerative disease. It's no wonder that health care in this country is in the midst of a major crisis.

At the beginning of this chapter, I noted how diet plays a substantial role in maintaining acid-alkaline balance. Everything you eat and drink either promotes or interferes with the balance of acids and alkalis in your body, and unfortunately, the standard American diet has a high proportion of acidifying foods. Even more unfortunate is the fact that so much of the available drinking water—which, in its purest form, is very alkalizing—is contaminated with acidic toxins.

The way out of this predicament is twofold. First, you must adjust your diet so that it supports acid-alkaline balance, and Chapter 7 provides plenty of nutritional guidance for this purpose. Second, and just as important, you should drink healthy, pure water that will not only bolster your body's acid-alkaline balance, but also fight the related problem of chronic dehydration. The next chapter turns to the primary subject of this book, ionized water, and explains how it is an ideal way to hydrate and alkalize your body.

3

The Ionized Water Solution

rinking purified water probably does not strike you as a novel idea, but it's a relatively recent health trend. In response to new information about the true quality of tap water, the twenty-first century has seen significant growth in the consumer market for bottled water as well as other water filtration and purification methods. People want to protect themselves from the harmful acidic chemicals and pollutants that flow out of their kitchen faucets, and mineral water, spring water, and alkalized water are some of the more popular go-to solutions.

Still, there's an even better—but mostly overlooked—answer to H_2O acidity and impurity. Ionized water, which possesses the same properties as the glacier-fed bodies of water in several mountainous regions, is superior to other kinds of water in terms of pH value, mineral content, and proper hydrating capability. And thanks to various technological advancements of the past century, you don't have to travel to the Himalayas in order to drink the purest water possible. Water can be ionized in your kitchen any time you need to quench your thirst, and every glass you drink comes with a host of health benefits. This chapter will introduce you to one of the most important discoveries in the fields of science and alternative health in recent decades. As you will see, ionized water is an effective remedy for chronic dehydration, acid-alkaline imbalance, and a number of other ailments.

IT BEGAN WITH THE HUNZA, IT ENDS IN YOUR HOME

Although the ionized water advocated in this book is produced with an electrolyzing device (see page 33), its health-enhancing properties are also found in nature. In fact, it was the study of the water of Hunza—a tiny region tucked away in the Himalayas of northwest Pakistan—that made scientists search for a way to reproduce it for the masses. The Hunza people have been renowned for their excellent health and longevity for nearly a century, as they generally live past the age of 100 free of bone loss, tooth decay, and degenerative diseases such as heart disease and cancer. Indeed, when asked for the secret to his people's vibrant health, a Hunza king replied, "It's the water."

This claim is backed by sound scientific research initiated by Dr. Henri Coanda, a Romanian known mainly for his work in the fields of fluid dynamics and aeronautics. Dr. Coanda spent six decades examining the Hunza people's glacier-fed drinking water to identify its health-giving features. He observed that its *surface tension* was low, making the water "wetter" and highly absorbable (see page 31), as well as a clustered crystalline structure similar to that of human body fluids. This latter characteristic was particularly important, since it meant that the water was already compatible with the body's biological processes. It was truly "living water."

As additional scientists joined Dr. Coanda's research effort, they realized that the "living water" was found in other regions where people similarly enjoyed good health and long lives—the Andes Mountains, the Caucasus region of southwestern Asia, and the Shin-Chan region of China. They also pinpointed more of this water's distinguishing characteristics, including an alkaline pH, an abundance of minerals, a high concentration of active hydrogen, and antioxidizing potential. The logical next step was to look for ways in which this water could be recreated and made available to people around the world.

For this task, scientists looked to the work of a British chemist and physicist, Michael Faraday, who invented the first electrolyzing apparatus in the nineteenth century. The device did not receive much acclaim during Faraday's lifetime, but it was groundbreaking in that it successfully separated water into its hydrogen and oxygen components. The invention took on new relevance in the early twentieth century as Russian scientists began experimenting with electrolysis. The methods that emerged from their testing were adapted by researchers in Japan to produce the first unit capable of simulating ionization by electrically "splitting" water molecules. The water was divided into acidic and alkaline water, filtered into separate chambers, and then closely studied by the scientists, who observed its remarkable resemblance to Hunza water in structure, chemical makeup, and healthful attributes.

A number of experiments were conducted before ionized water was finally deemed safe enough to test on humans. Scientists in Japan first administered alkaline ionized water to plants and animals, and noted positive changes in the health of both. They were especially encouraged by these results because neither plants nor animals are subject to the placebo effect—a factor that must normally be considered in scientific experiments because it may influence results. Eventually, they were able to prove that ionized water was not only safe for human consumption, but also highly advantageous in terms of improving health. Ionized water was thus deemed "functional water technology."

In 1958, large commercial ionizers were manufactured in Japan, followed closely thereafter by smaller residential units. Two years later, Japanese physicians and agricultural researchers founded an institute dedicated to the continued study of ionized water. By the mid-1960s, ionizers were used in Japanese hospitals and considered to be legitimate medical devices. It is estimated that, since then, over thirty million Japanese people have used water ionizers for the purpose of improving their health.

The use of water ionizers has expanded globally over the last several decades, introduced to South Korea in the 1970s and to the United States in 1985. The ionizer was tested by an independent research team in Los Angeles according to standards set by the Food and Drug Administration (FDA), and ultimately found to be safe and capable of producing higher-quality drinking water. A number of physicians and members of the American general public began to use ionizers for personal use in the 1990s, but they continue to be more widely employed in other countries such as Australia, Canada, New Zealand, and various Asian and European nations. This is mainly because most Americans are unaware that ionized water is a readily available resource that can be produced in their own home. As you will see, the ionization process is simple, quick, and convenient.

WHAT IS IONIZATION?

In order to better understand what ionized water actually is, you should have a basic understanding of the process of ionization. Let's start with a chemical formula you surely know—H_2O. This chemical symbol for water represents its composition. It is two parts hydrogen and one part oxygen. In more scientific terms, this means that one molecule of water consists of two hydrogen atoms and one oxygen atom.

Let's examine these hydrogen and oxygen atoms more closely in order to understand the significance of the chemical reaction for water. The makeup of a hydrogen atom is very simple. If you were to view one under a molecular microscope, you would see that its nucleus contains a single *proton*, a positively charged particle. Revolving around the nucleus is a single *electron*, a particle with a negative charge. In comparison, the makeup of an oxygen atom is a little more complex; its nucleus contains eight protons, and orbiting around the nucleus are eight electrons. The fact that oxygen has paired electrons (an even number) and hydrogen has only one electron (an odd number) is significant, as Dr. Hidemitsu Hayashi, Director of the Water Institute of Japan, has recognized: "The single hydrogen electron and the eight electrons of oxygen are the key to the chemistry of life because this is where hydrogen and oxygen atoms combine to form a water molecule, or split to form ions."

What Dr. Hayashi is referring to here is the process of *ionization*, which occurs when an atom or group of atoms gains a positive or negative charge during various chemical reactions. Ionization can happen in one of two ways. An atom, usually already unstable due to an odd number of electrons, can lose electrons, or it can bond itself to another atom or molecule. The electrically charged particle that results is called an *ion*. The loss of electrons from an atom or molecule forms positively charged ions known as *cations*, while the gain of electrons forms negatively charged ions known as *anions*.

In the chemical reaction for water, it is hydrogen that is ionized, since its single electron makes it unstable and more reactive. The byproducts of ionization in this case are *hydrogen ions* and *hydroxyl ions*. Hydrogen ions, represented with the symbol H+, are the positively charged particles that form when hydrogen's single electron is lost. As you will recall from Chapter 2, water with a high concentration of hydrogen (H+) ions is acidic, so it will increase your body's pH level when you drink it. *Hydroxyl ions*, on the other hand, form when a whole hydrogen atom joins to a whole oxygen atom, creating a negatively charged particle represented by the symbol OH-. Unlike hydrogen ions, a high concentration of hydroxyl ions in water makes it very alkalizing. In fact, hydroxyl ions have been considered a basic building block of life, containing life-giving energy that they are able to donate to any and all compatible atoms in every living organism, including human beings.

As you can see, ionization is a process that occurs naturally, and all drinking water is ionized to some degree. Still, it isn't enough. The water I discuss in this book is ionized through a mild electrolyzing process, which separates it into its acidic (hydrogen ions) and alkaline (hydroxyl ions) components to maximize the water's health-enhancing properties. In other words, technology has made it possible to reproduce the process of ionization in order to maximize its effects. The special characteristics of the water that is created are detailed in the next section.

THE IONIZED WATER DIFFERENCE

By now, you're aware that ionization produces water that is extremely alkalizing due to a high concentration of hydroxyl ions. Alkaline water helps to balance the body's pH and eliminate acid wastes from cells, tissues, and organs. Moreover, due to the high concentration of hydroxyl ions, alkaline water contains life-supporting energy that makes it an effective *antioxidant,* a protective substance that prevents potentially harmful reactions from occurring in the body. (See Chapter 4 for more about ionized water as an antioxidant.)

In recent years, the benefits of alkaline water have been more widely appreciated, especially since the acidic contents of tap water have come under public scrutiny. Many people have taken to drinking filtered water, mineralized water, and bottled alkaline water in an effort to avoid harmful contaminants and hydrate their bodies with more purifying H_2O. In consideration of the dangers of acid-alkaline imbalance, others add alkalizing drops and baking soda to their drinking water to increase its pH. While these methods may improve the water's alkalinity, they do not come close to ionized water in terms of health benefits. Bottled alkaline water, for example, loses much of its antioxidant strength in the time it takes to be bottled, distributed to stores, and then finally purchased. In addition, adding alkalizing substances (such as chemical drops and baking soda) to water does not fundamentally change the water itself. Unlike ionized water, the structure of simply "alkalized" water remains the same.

The key to improving water's overall quality is *electrolysis,* the process that takes place in a water ionizer. In other words, science is used to reproduce a substance that is naturally occurring. By receiving an electrical charge, the water is fundamentally changed and given the following properties:

- **Clustered structure.** Ionized water is smaller in structure than other types of H_2O, composed of a cluster of four to six water molecules (as compared to the usual ten to fifteen). This significantly smaller size allows your body to absorb it more easily and efficiently, forcing toxins out of your cells and tissues. (See inset on page 32.) Additionally, the angle of the molecular bonds between the oxygen and hydrogen atoms improves oxygenation of the body.

- **Electrical charge.** Ionized water is the only type of water capable of holding an electrical charge, which is why it's so vitalizing and conductive. Because of this electrical charge, ionized water is extremely efficient when it comes to transporting nutrients and oxygen to the body's cells.

- **Hexagonal shape.** Unlike other types of water, ionized water molecules are shaped like hexagons, having six sides. This distinct shape allows the water to move quickly throughout the body and carry more nutrients and oxygen. This, in turn, enhances internal cleansing, metabolic activity, cellular function, and energy.

- **Hydrogen bonds.** Ionized water is primarily composed of hydrogen bonds, which enhance and support all of the vital functions that occur in your body at the cellular level.

- **Leftward spin.** While the electrons in regular water molecules orbit in a counterclockwise (rightward) direction, the electrons of ionized water molecules spin to the left. This spin indicates that ionized water contains energy, meaning that it is active, vitalizing, and, therefore, able to boost your well-being.

- **Low surface tension.** Surface tension is the term used to describe the tendency of liquids to molecularly "gel," which is why many objects are able to float on water's surface. When water has a low surface tension, the molecules are more elastic and less cohesive, which allows the H_2O to flow quickly throughout your body and effortlessly penetrate cells and tissues.

- **Positive charge.** The positive charge of ionized water enables it to significantly improve cell-to-cell communication, a benefit no other kind of water can supply.

- **Purity.** Ionized water is considered to be pure because it does not contain the negative electromagnetic frequency imprints found in most water, especially the recycled sewage water of many municipalities. These toxic imprints are eliminated during the ionization process.

These characteristics are inherent to the H_2O found in regions with pure water sources, such as Hunza. However, technology is required in order to return our water to its more natural state. Water ionizers both electrolyze and filter H_2O, which makes them the ultimate one-two punch of water filtration methods as well as one of the best investments you can make for your health.

HOW WATER IONIZERS WORK

A water ionizer is not your typical water filter. Water distillers and reverse osmosis (RO) filters have become popular in recent years, but, as most health professionals know, they are not effective solutions to water acidity and contamination. In fact, drinking distilled water can be more harmful than good for you, since it is stripped of vital minerals. And although reverse osmosis filters may remove

Agre, Aquaporins, and Ionized H₂O

As you read on page 30, the micro-clustering that occurs during the ionization process results in water that is deeply hydrating. To understand why, you should be familiar with the research of Dr. Peter Agre, who won the Nobel Prize in Chemistry in 2003 for discovering how water penetrates human cells.

Scientists had previously believed that water moved through cell membranes much in the same way water leaks through a cloth. However, Dr. Agre found that H_2O actually enters by way of small pores called *aquaporins,* which are made of proteins and extend all the way through the cell wall. Aquaporins selectively conduct water molecules in and out of cells while simultaneously preventing the passage of ions and other soluble materials, including fluoride and impurities found in tap water. Amazingly, only one water molecule is able to enter through the cell wall at a time, which is important to the study of ionized water. Since the process of ionization reduces water clusters to one-third of their normal size, the water is much closer in size to that of a single water molecule. Therefore, they easily pass through the aquaporins, hydrating the cells and tissues.

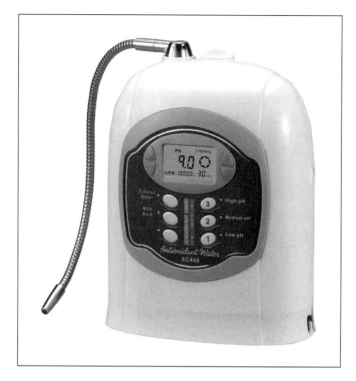

Water Ionizer

many toxic chemicals from the water, they are very wasteful and do not significantly diminish the water's acidifying quality. As I mentioned earlier, the key to drastically improving the quality of drinking water is electrolysis. The electrolyzing process performed by water ionizers changes the structure of the water and separates it into its alkaline and acidic forms. Let's briefly explore how water ionizers work.

It's important to first mention that water ionizers manufactured today are easy to install and small enough to fit on a kitchen countertop. (See Chapter 8 for a consumer's guide to water ionizers.) The illustration above gives a general idea of what one of these units looks like.

Typically, ionizers also have adjustable settings, so you can choose the level of alkalinity or acidity of the water produced before you start—the generated water may have a pH as high as 10.0 or as low as 2.0.

When you first turn on the faucet, the tap water is redirected by a special attachment that hooks onto the faucet, and flows through a plastic hose into the ionizer. Once inside the ionizer unit, the water passes through an activated filter that removes chemicals and other pollutants. From here, the water flows into a chamber that contains platinum-coated titanium electrodes with positive and negative charges. It is inside this chamber that the water is electrolyzed.

Two separate processes take place during electrolysis. First, positive ions (cations) in the water accumulate around the negatively charged electrodes, which produces highly alkaline, micro-cluster water. This water, which is intended for drinking, flows out of a faucet-like attachment on the ionizer unit. Second, and at the same time, the negative ions (anions) in the water gather around the positively charged electrodes to produce acidic water, which empties out into the sink through a separate hose. As you will read in Chap-

Stomach Acids and Alkaline Water

Whenever I lecture about the benefits of alkaline ionized water, invariably I am asked about stomach acid. Usually the question is this: Doesn't the acid in my stomach neutralize the alkaline water and negate its benefits?

The answer to this question is no. Despite television commercials that suggest otherwise, our stomachs are usually empty. Strong stomach acids are produced only when food is present, especially acidic food high in fat and protein. Water, therefore, does not stimulate the secretion of stomach acids, but instead simply passes through the stomach into the small intestine, where it is absorbed.

Even when acids are present in the stomach, the benefits of drinking alkaline ionized water are not undermined. This is because the water also enters the bloodstream and is transported to cells, tissues, and organs. In addition, the stomach offsets the acids it produces by making an equal amount of alkalis, which are then discharged into the bloodstream. So, although the alkaline ionized water may be neutralized in the stomach, there is still a net gain of alkalinity for the body.

ter 6, this acidic water has a variety of external uses, including cleaning and skin care.

The entire process—starting from the moment you turn on the faucet and ending when the water flows out of its respective attachment—takes only one or two minutes. Best of all, once the unit is installed, you only need to turn on your faucet in order to use it. What could be simpler? A household water ionizer allows you to drink water in its purest form any time you want.

CONCLUSION

Arguably, ionized water is our most overlooked tool in the struggle against the related issues of chronic dehydration and acid-alkaline imbalance. Drinking water that has been electrolyzed and filtered in an ionizer is the equivalent of drinking the fresh, glacier-fed water of the Hunza region, where the vast majority of people enjoy a long life free of chronic disease. Thanks to the innovative work of scientists around the world, it is now possible for anyone to drink water that is highly alkaline, rich in nutrients and minerals, and full of antioxidants—without having to leave home. The structural and chemical properties of ionized water, both acidic and alkaline, make it a unique type of H_2O that can be a real asset to your health. Consuming alkaline ionized water is effective for preventing and treating disease, and the next chapter looks at the two main driving forces behind its health-sustaining capabilities—alkalinity and antioxidant strength.

4

Two Key Features of Ionized Drinking Water

As you learned in the previous chapter, alkaline ionized water is identical to the "living water" of glacial streams and many other natural water sources. Such water is said to be "living" because of its structural and chemical similarity to fluids found in the vascular pathways—the channels through which nutrients and other vital substances are transported—of both plants and animals, including humans. In other words, living water is suited to our biological needs and processes; it promotes optimal wellness.

The life-supporting quality of living water, and thus alkaline ionized water, is demonstrated in a variety of ways (see Chapter 5), but most of these are rooted in two key features. Ionized water acts as a potent antioxidant, and due to its high alkaline pH value, it improves the oxygenation of the body. Drinking alkaline ionized water equips your system with disease-fighting ability and an enriched oxygen supply, which enables your body to maintain balance, function properly, and generally remain in a state of good health. Notably, antioxidants and adequate oxygen levels also go a long way in the prevention of cancer, as cancerous cells thrive in oxygen-deficient environments where they can roam unchecked. This chapter provides an overview of the two overriding benefits of ionized water—its alkalizing and antioxidizing strength—to help you better understand how and why drinking ionized water can alleviate and even thwart the conditions discussed in future chapters.

ANTIOXIDANTS AND IONIZED WATER

It has already been mentioned that an *antioxidant* is a molecule or substance that prevents the occurrence of potentially harmful chemical reactions in the body. More specifically, antioxidants hinder the process of *oxidation,* which is caused by unstable, highly reactive atoms or molecules known as oxidizers, or *free radicals.* Free radicals appear in the body as a normal byproduct of bodily processes such as digestion and respiration, or form as a result of various medications, smoking, or overexposure to environmental pollution and sunlight. Chemically unstable due to an insufficient number of electrons in their outer orbit, free radicals scour the body unrestricted looking for electrons to "steal." In doing so, they damage nearly every piece of matter with which they come into contact until they successfully take an electron from another atom or molecule. Over time, the total damage inflicted can be widespread and severe. To give a more concrete picture, oxidation is like having a person loose in your house with a small sledgehammer hitting everything in sight. Although each individual blow of the hammer causes minimal damage, before long, your whole house will be destroyed. When free radicals latch onto healthy cells, for instance, they can cause major damage to tissues and organs, resulting in conditions such as cardiovascular disease, neurological disorders, and type 2 diabetes, along with many others.

This is where antioxidants enter the picture, and their function is exactly as their name implies—they prevent oxidation. Whereas oxidizers, or free radicals, are missing electrons, antioxidants have an extra electron in their outer orbit that they are able to "donate" without becoming unstable themselves. Therefore, when an oxidizer and an antioxidant meet, there is an electron exchange that effectively neutralizes the oxidizer's destructive potential. The free radical is stabilized, and further oxidative damage is halted. With enough antioxidants, damage in the body can even be reversed.

The electron exchange between an antioxidant and a free radical is referred to as an oxidation-reduction, or redox, reaction. Simply put, reduction is the opposite of oxidation—electrons are removed during an oxidative reaction and added during a redox reaction. The addition of an electron to an atom or molecule means that energy is being transferred to the molecule that is being reduced, or neutralized. So if a substance has reducing potential (the ability to protect against oxidation), it is capable of donating energy to the body via the extra electrons it contains. This ability is determined by a measurement called *oxidation-reduction potential* (ORP), also known as redox potential. Redox potential is quantified using the *millivolt* (mV), which is the equivalent of one thousandth of a volt. A measurement of zero is neutral, positive readings (numbers over zero) indicate oxidizing potential, and negative readings (numbers below zero) indicate reducing potential—the power to act as an antioxidant.

Although the body produces antioxidants naturally, its ability to do so weakens with age, and it may not produce enough to offset an abundance of free radicals. For this reason, it's important to supplement your body's resources with a nutritious diet of foods and beverages rich in antioxidants. (See inset on page 40.) Still, there's no other substance that compares to alkaline ionized water when it comes to redox potential. As opposed to tap water, which has an ORP measurement of +400 mV to +500 mV, and regular mineral water, which shows a reading of +200 mV, alkaline ionized water has a remarkable redox potential of –250 to –350 mV. In other words, whereas tap water is oxidizing, alkaline ionized water is an antioxidant—it is plentiful in extra electrons with which it can counteract free radicals, thereby protecting cells, tissues, and organs from infection and disease.

The superiority of alkaline ionized water to nutritional antioxidants is derived from the electrolysis process through which it is produced. When water is electrolyzed, its molecules receive an excess of electrons, enabling them to stabilize the free radicals they encounter. In addition, as you may recall from Chapter 3, electrolysis reduces the size of clusters in water molecules. A more compact size in combination with a lower molecular weight means that the water can travel throughout the body at a more efficient rate, reaching all of your cells and tissues more quickly than other substances.

The molecular weights of antioxidants commonly found in food sources—for instance, beta-carotene, vitamin C, and vitamin E—are nearly nine times heavier than that of alkaline ionized water. Therefore, they do not permeate cells as easily or rapidly.

The high redox potential of alkaline ionized water is unmatched by any other type of water. Every time you drink a glass of this H_2O, you neutralize dangerous free radicals, in turn reinforcing your body's immune system. This is crucial for treating and preventing a number of conditions, many of which will be discussed in the next chapter. Now, we turn to the other paramount property of alkaline ionized water—its positive influence on bodily oxygenation.

Eliminating Free Radicals With Your Food

Because of the importance of antioxidants to your well-being, leading health organizations such as the American Heart Association and American Cancer Society recommend that you follow a diet plentiful in antioxidant-rich foods. Although alkaline ionized water is a more potent antioxidant overall, eating foods that contain significant amounts of beta-carotene, selenium, vitamin C, and vitamin E will help to further fortify your immune system against disease and infection. Below is a list of some of the top food sources of antioxidants in order of the amount they contain, according to a recent study by the United States Department of Agriculture (USDA).

- Beans (red, kidney, pinto, and black)
- Berries (blackberries, blueberries, cranberries, raspberries, strawberries)
- Artichoke hearts, cooked
- Prunes
- Apples (with peel, particularly Gala, Granny Smith, and Red Delicious)
- Nuts, particularly hazelnuts, pecans, and walnuts
- Cherries
- Plums
- Russet potatoes
- Spices such as cinnamon, oregano, and ground cloves

ALKALINITY, "VITAMIN O," AND IONIZED WATER

Along with water, oxygen is the body's primary source of life. It makes up approximately 65 percent of the elements found in your body, including your blood, cells, tissues, organs, and skin. It is also intimately involved in nearly all physiological activities, fueling cellular energy factories (the mitochondria) as the main component of *adenosine triphosphate* (*ATP*)—the body's energy currency. Oxygen is one of your body's chief lines of defense against harmful microorganisms, which is why O_2 deficiency has been linked to common infections as well as serious illnesses like cancer. In addition, sleep problems, mood disorders, high blood pressure, and even Alzheimer's disease may be connected to a low supply of oxygen in the body. For these reasons and many others, doctors often refer to oxygen as "vitamin O," a name that accurately conveys its importance to your health and well-being.

However, the body's oxygen levels drop when the pH of the blood becomes too acidic. Acidity increases the thickness of the blood, interfering with the circulation and assimilation of oxygen, which is carried and delivered to cells and tissues by way of the hemoglobin. The scientific term for the capacity of the blood to deliver oxygen on the cellular level is the *oxygen-hemoglobin dissociation curve,* and even a slight change in pH can affect this capability. The blood might be saturated with oxygen, but unless its pH is alkaline, the oxygen will not be released—or dissociated—from the hemoglobin. When this capability is prevented or impaired, cells lose the ability to repair themselves and eliminate waste, which can cause you to experience fatigue and perhaps other symptoms as well (see inset on page 42). Soon, bodily tissues will begin to feel the damaging effects of oxygen deficiency as they become more susceptible to infection by invading microorganisms. Cancer is just one of the chronic degenerative diseases that may develop, a topic that receives a more detailed explanation on page 45.

The relationship between oxygenation and pH balance is one of the chief reasons why drinking alkalized water is so beneficial—you are essentially filling your body with its two basic requirements, pure H$_2$O and oxygen, simultaneously. In addition, as you may recall from Chapter 3, the particular shape and structure of the water's molecular makeup makes it conducive to oxygenation of the body, since it is easily transported by the blood and absorbed by the cells. The electrical charge the water receives as a result of electrolysis also increases its efficiency in penetrating cells and tissues and providing them with vital materials. Coupled with its alkalinity, the structural and chemical properties of alkaline ionized water will help boost your body's oxygen levels every time you drink it, thereby reducing your risk of numerous medical conditions such as the ones outlined in the next section.

Do You Have a "Vitamin O" Deficiency?

Oxygen is essential not only for survival but also for optimal functioning of the body. In a state of rest, the average adult requires approximately one cup of oxygen per minute. During periods of rigorous activity, the amount of needed oxygen increases to nearly two gallons per minute. Clearly, it's critical that you have an adequate supply at all times.

Unfortunately, due to the high rate of acidosis among the American population, many people suffer from oxygen deficiency without knowing it. Here are some of the most common signs of an insufficient O$_2$ level:

- Circulation problems
- Depression
- Digestive problems
- Dizziness
- Fatigue
- Infections

- Irritability
- Memory loss
- Muscle aches
- Poor concentration
- Susceptibility to illnesses such as colds and the flu

You should consult your health-care provider if you experience any number of these symptoms. A blood test may be used to determine the level of oxygen in your body. Oxygen-rich blood is bright red in appearance, while a dull red color indicates an inadequate oxygen level.

OXYGEN AND YOUR HEALTH

Now that you know how acid-alkaline balance and oxygenation are related not only to each other but also to good health, it's time to take a closer look at the medical issues that may arise when alkalinity and, therefore, proper oxygen levels are not maintained. Immunity, cognitive function, cardiovascular health, and the body's ability to fight cancer are all affected, and their relationship to sufficient oxygenation—and, by extension, acid-alkaline balance—is discussed below.

Immune Function

There are a number of factors that contribute to healthy immune function, including a nutritious, well-balanced diet, plenty of exercise and sleep, and effective stress management. But the best protective shield against harmful bacteria, fungi, parasites, and viruses is an adequate oxygen supply. When your body is in an *aerobic* (oxygen-rich) state, it is better able to defend itself against an onslaught of microbe invaders, as they cannot survive in well-oxygenated environments for very long. Oxygen-rich blood is a staple of a healthy immune system— microorganisms will simply weaken and die instead of attacking cells.

An *anaerobic* (oxygen-deficient) internal environment, however, allows disease-causing agents to thrive and wreak havoc on your cells and tissues. The vast majority of people who suffer from serious health conditions are usually in a chronic anaerobic state. In fact, it is possible to reverse many diseases simply by returning the body to an aerobic state, which, of course, also means restoring pH balance.

Brain Function

Your brain requires approximately 20 percent of all the oxygen you take in each day. When not enough O_2 is available, an array of symptoms will soon appear, ranging from poor concentration, forgetfulness, and other cognitive impairments to mood swings, restlessness, and feelings of anxiety or depression. Sleep apnea may also develop due to an insufficient amount of oxygen reaching the brain. Conversely, research has shown that when the body's oxygen supply is elevated, mental functions such as memory are enhanced.

Moreover, recent studies have suggested that a lack of oxygen may be one of the main causes of Alzheimer's disease. One such study is the 2006 experiment at the Brain Research Center at the University of British Columbia in Canada, in which a research team analyzed the effects of varying oxygen levels on the brains of mice. They discovered that an oxygen deficiency triggered the BACE1 gene, which is connected to Alzheimer's in humans, to produce more amyloid beta plaque, protein deposits that are linked to the development of the disease. Based on these findings, the scientists concluded that there is a correlation between proper oxygen levels and Alzheimer's risk.

Contrary to popular belief, breathing pure oxygen is not a safe or efficient way to improve the function and oxygen level of the brain—doing so may even cause damage. The best way to ensure that the brain receives the oxygen it needs is to keep the body in a state of pH balance through diet and water intake, as well as to engage in aerobic exercise.

Cardiovascular Health

Like every other muscle in your body, the heart works efficiently only if it receives an adequate amount of oxygen. And the heart requires more oxygen than other muscles, since it is directly responsible for the delivery of O_2 to your organs by pumping blood. Because of the integral role the heart plays in the distribution of oxygen, it's very common for doctors to monitor heart patients' blood oxygen levels. Administering oxygen to heart attack and stroke victims is a conventional medical practice, and long-term oxygen therapy is frequently used to treat people suffering from chronic heart disease.

Alkaline ionized water is an ideal remedy for heart problems stemming from low oxygen levels, since chronic dehydration is often tied to cardiovascular disorders such as high blood pressure and high cholesterol. In other words, drinking alkaline ionized water allows you to simultaneously hydrate *and* oxygenate your body, thereby equipping it with the two most essential ingredients for maintaining a healthy heart.

Cancer Prevention

Cancer is one of the leading causes of death in the United States, second only to heart disease, and feared more than any other. Each year, more than one million Americans are diagnosed with some form of cancer, and over half a million more die from it. Internal factors such as genetic and hormonal abnormalities, as well as external factors like radiation, toxins, and infectious agents have all been named as possible causes of cancer. However, according to German physician Otto Heinrich Warburg, there is only one cause, which is "the replacement of the respiration of oxygen in normal body cells by a fermentation of sugar." In the view of Warburg, a winner of the Nobel Prize in Medicine, the proliferation of cancerous cells is directly related to low oxygen levels because, as he himself discovered, abnormal cells flourish in low-oxygen environments.

The growth and spread of cancer cells, Dr. Warburg concluded, can be attributed to a process called *glycolysis,* which occurs when oxygen-deprived cells revert to a "primitive" or unhealthy state and begin to derive their energy from glucose (via fermentation) rather than oxygen. Today, the mainstream medical establishment acknowledges that cancer cells generate energy through glycolysis but have not yet accepted Warburg's theory that glycolysis is also the primary cause of cancer's development. However, cancer detection technology like positron emission tomography (PET) scans often involves tracking the body's use of glucose.

Still, Dr. Warburg's work has led to widespread recognition of the interconnectedness of cancer, oxygen, and acid-alkaline balance. In addition to his research on glycolysis, he wrote extensively about the relationship between oxygen and pH, which he observed was directly proportional: The higher the concentration of oxygen molecules, the higher (more alkaline) the pH, and vice versa. His findings have enabled a number of scientists and cancer physicians specializing in alternative health to develop oxygen-based treatment methods and therapies.

Yet, it is easier to prevent cancer than it is to treat it. This is where alkaline ionized water comes in. You already know that the high alkalinity of ionized H_2O will at once raise your body's oxygen levels and work to restore acid-alkaline balance, and both of these healthful effects will support cancer resistance. On top of this, alkaline ionized water also helps to prevent unhealthy fermentation by reducing the amount of *metabolites*, the potentially harmful byproducts of digestion, in the gastrointestinal tract. By impeding the fermentation process, alkaline ionized H_2O also hinders glycolysis—the chemical reaction that spurs cancer growth. The anticancer properties of alkaline ionized water will be explained in further detail in Chapter 5.

CONCLUSION

Although good health depends on a number of factors, alkaline ionized water provides some of the most basic and important ones. Its effectiveness as an antioxidant in combination with its high pH value gives the water its vitalizing and disease-fighting strength. Equipped with these key features, it works to neutralize free radicals, boost acid-alkaline balance, and oxygenate the body, all of which create an environment adverse to harmful microorganisms. For this reason, drinking alkaline ionized H_2O can be a powerful tool in reducing the risk of cognitive dysfunction (including Alzheimer's disease), heart disease, and even cancer. In other words, alkaline ionized water is truly "living water," and its antioxidizing potency and high pH are two major reasons why. This knowledge is essential for understanding the other health benefits of alkaline ionized water, which either directly or indirectly stem from the characteristics discussed in this chapter. When it comes to preventing disease and maintaining good health, drinking ionized H_2O can make all the difference.

5

The Health Benefits of Alkaline Ionized Water

As the late Dr. Mu Shik Jhon, a Korean scientist and one of the world's leading experts on ionized water, once wrote, "All water is not created equal and it is the structure of water within our bodies that ultimately determines health or sickness." Alkaline ionized water, as you now know, promotes health and works against sickness—it hydrates, alkalizes, and oxygenates the body, all while acting as a powerful antioxidant. Its distinctive properties, such as small cluster size and hexagonal structure, are matched by no other type of water except the kind found in regions like Hunza, where drinking water is derived directly from glacial streams. Alkaline ionized water is "living" and can help *you* live a longer, healthier life. This chapter looks at the major diseases and debilitating conditions that alkaline ionized water may both prevent and alleviate. Most of these conditions are serious health dangers like cancer and type 2 diabetes, which afflict increasingly large portions of our population.

ALLERGIES

In order to understand how alkaline ionized water relates to allergies, you should first be familiar with *histamine*, a brain chemical that, among other functions, is responsible for producing immune responses and thirst signals. Histamine is released when a physiological need arises, whether for food, water, or defense against a potentially harmful substance. The chemical is also released during an allergic reaction, which is an immune response triggered by a substance such as nuts or ragweed that should not pose a danger. This is why allergies are considered autoimmune disorders and treated with antihistamine medications to control and counteract allergic reactions.

However, antihistamines can also cause dehydration by interfering with the thirst mechanism. This fact has led several doctors, including Dr. Batmanghelidj (introduced in Chapter 1) to the conclusion that allergies can be treated by increasing water intake. Hydrating the body inhibits the excess production and release of histamine, thus halting the occurrence of allergic reactions. According to Dr. Batmanghelidj, "This relationship of water to histamine has been demonstrated in several animal experiments. It is now physiologically apparent that water by itself has very strong antihistaminic properties." Simply put, increasing water intake can alleviate, if not eliminate, allergies and asthma.

Because of ionized water's superior absorbability, it stands to reason that its antihistamine effects are also enhanced. Moreover, the alkalinity and antioxidizing strength of the water makes it more capable of suppressing allergies, which often go hand in hand with over-acidification and low levels of alkalizing minerals in the body. In fact, these conditions are often the root cause of allergies in the first place, as they reduce immunity. Alkaline ionized water bolsters immune function because it contains ionic calcium, a mineral that counteracts toxins and controls acidity, in turn increasing the body's resistance to allergies.

The healing power of alkaline ionized H_2O has been extensively studied, tested, and observed by a number of physicians such as Dr. Kuninaka Hironaga, the head of Kuninaka Hospital in Japan, who experienced the water's curative effects firsthand. He reported, "Ever since I began to consume antioxidant water, [my] allergy has recovered." Dr. Hironaga also started one of his patients on an alkaline ionized water regimen to treat his severe allergy. The trial was met with success, and no relapse occurred. Since then, scientists and doctors have found several other allergy cases that respond well to alkaline ionized water.

ARTHRITIS AND JOINT PAIN

Arthritis and joint pain are two of the most frequent health complaints in the United States. According to the Centers for Disease Control and Prevention, the number of people suffering from this disabling disease has risen from 46 million to 50 million people in the last four years, which means that approximately 22 percent of the population is afflicted with it. In the vast majority of cases, both rheumatoid arthritis and osteoarthritis are caused by two factors—chronic acidosis and chronic dehydration. Let's examine each of these factors separately and address how alkaline ionized water can solve the problem.

When the body is in an overly acidic state for a prolonged period, *uric acid* accumulates in the bloodstream. Uric acid is a normal byproduct of nitrogen metabolism and an inevitable result of a diet high in acidic foods like meat, poultry, fish, and alcohol. Because uric acid cannot be destroyed or safely stored in the body, it must be eliminated through urination. When the body is properly balanced, this can be done easily. However, acidosis causes excessive buildup of uric acid that is much more difficult to completely purge from your system, and eventually, the buildup becomes solidified as uric acid crystals. These crystals are deposited in the tissues and joints, leading to destroyed cartilage, joint irritation, swelling, and even severe pain—the primary symptoms of a form of arthritis known as gout.

Dr. Batmanghelidj has pointed to chronic dehydration as a leading cause of arthritis and joint pain. This is due to the fact that water lubricates the surfaces of cartilage. Thus, when the body experiences a water deficiency, the amount of water between the joints is reduced, forcing them to rub against each other. This constant friction produces joint damage, paving the way for arthritis.

Alkaline ionized water acts as both remedy and prevention tool when it comes to arthritis. This, of course, is due to its alkalizing and hydrating capabilities. Its high alkaline pH can dramatically lower the level of acidity in the body, helping to shrink the amount of uric acid crystals until they are completely eradicated. In addition, alkaline ionized water penetrates cells more quickly, hydrating the body and lubricating the joints more efficiently. Hydration and proper acid-alkaline balance, both of which are achieved by drinking alkaline ionized H_2O regularly, will certainly reverse the progression of arthritis and joint pain.

CANCER

A discussion of alkaline ionized water's health benefits is not complete without mention of its potential as an anticancer agent. Cancer affects millions of lives every year, and despite the US government's "war on cancer" declared in 1971, the incidence of the disease has skyrocketed. Today, over 1.5 million people are diagnosed with some form of cancer each year, and millions more either have a history of cancer or are currently receiving treatment for the disease. Having specialized in cancer treatment for several years, I've come to realize that successfully dealing with the illness requires a comprehensive, multilayered approach that takes all possible factors into account. Unfortunately, most conventional cancer doctors focus solely on "slash and burn" treatment methods, which typically consist of surgery followed by intensive chemotherapy and/or radiation therapy. These therapies attack cancerous cells and tumors but do little to address the many underlying and interrelated causes of cancer. Based on my years of clinical experience, I believe that truly effective cancer care not only targets the cancer itself, but also includes:

- Bolstering immune function through proper diet and the use of appropriate nutritional supplementation.

- Dealing with any unresolved psychological issues that may be creating anxiety or stress.

- Stimulating the body's ability to eliminate toxins through various detoxification methods, such as organic diets or internal cleanses using bentonite clay or chlorella, medicinal substances that promote a healthy colon and bowel.

To accomplish these goals, a treatment program that incorporates a variety of methods must be followed, taking the patient's individual needs into careful consideration. Such an approach allows for a greater chance of recovery and long-term survival than that which is achieved through conventional medicine alone.

There is no "magic bullet" for cancer, and ionized water is no exception. However, I believe that daily consumption of alkaline ionized water can be effective in the prevention of and recovery from cancer. As explained in Chapter 4, two of the primary causes of cancer are an oxygen deficiency in cells and tissues—a breakthrough that earned Dr. Otto Warburg a Nobel Prize—and free radical damage. Alkaline ionized water at once boosts oxygenation and reduces oxidation, inhibiting unhealthy cells from ravaging the body. For this reason, ionized H_2O provides powerful resistance to the growth and proliferation of cancer, and two recent scientific studies clearly demonstrate this fact.

The first study analyzed the effects of "electrolyzed reduced water" (in other words, alkaline ionized water) on tumor *angiogenesis,* a term used to describe the development of blood vessels. Cancer cells spread and grow into tumors by developing blood vessels through which they can receive energizing substances such as glucose, which acts as cancer's primary fuel. These blood vessels also divert vital materials that normal cells require to stay healthy. This is why patients with advanced forms of cancer sometimes appear to be "wasting away." In a very real sense, they are—the cancerous blood vessels are depriving their bodies of the necessary sustenance. As such, stopping tumor angiogenesis is a principal goal of many cancer physicians, and, in recent years, a number of drug companies have begun to develop anti-angiogenic drugs for this purpose.

The study, which was published in the medical journal *Biological and Pharmaceutical Bulletin* in 2008, specifically focused on the body's production of vascular endothelial growth factor (VEGF), a substance that enables tumor angiogenesis. High oxidative stress (free radical damage) stimulates production of abnormal levels of VEGF, which then stimulates tumor angiogenesis with the aid of another substance known as ERK. Remarkably, the researchers found that alkaline ionized water deactivated ERK, thus preventing the production of VEGF and tumor angiogenesis.

Another study, collectively conducted by scientists at various medical universities in Japan, similarly demonstrated the anti-cancer properties of alkaline ionized water. They first tested its ability to effectively treat cancer by injecting mice with B16 melanoma cells, a type of cancer that occurs frequently in humans and is known for its high capacity for rapid *metastasis,* or growth. The mice were divided into control and test groups so that results could be accurately measured. In the test group, the researchers observed a significant delay in tumor growth and a much longer lifespan compared to the control group. Furthermore, the alkaline water prevented metastasis of the melanoma cancer cells by dramatically reducing their number after they were injected into the test group mice. The researchers also reported that the water drastically lessened the amount of oxidative stress present in the test group. In terms of cancer prevention, they found that alkaline ionized H_2O provided anticancer benefits to healthy mice, boosting their immune function.

The scientists concluded their report by asserting that "alkaline reduced water is expected to be effective for the various diseases resulting from low immunity and/or high reactive oxygen species as well as for the prevention of cancer." Alkaline ionized water has high pH, low ORP, and a significant concentration of minerals like magnesium and ionic calcium, traits that lend themselves well to cancer resistance. When combined with its ability to move throughout the body quickly and be easily absorbed by cells, alkaline ionized water is, as the researchers put it simply, "an ideal way to maintain health."

Based on these findings, the potential of alkaline ionized water to act as an anticancer agent is an exciting prospect. However, this does not mean that it's a *cure.* Alkaline ionized water fortifies your system and creates an internal environment conducive for healing, but it does not alone eradicate the disease. Rather, it allows positive shifts to occur in your body, leading to the reduction and even elimination of harmful symptoms and bodily conditions.

CARDIOVASCULAR DISEASE

Cardiovascular disease is a term that encompasses a range of conditions that affect the heart, two of which—high cholesterol and hypertension—are discussed later in this chapter (see pages 57 and 59). Although the name is often used interchangeably with *heart disease*, which covers heart defects as well as rhythm problems, cardiovascular disease specifically refers to conditions having to do with your blood vessels, such as narrowed or blocked arteries. Such conditions significantly increase the risk of serious health issues like heart attack, stroke, aneurysms, and heart failure.

Water intake can dramatically affect the consistency of your blood, which is more than 80 percent water. For instance, your red blood cells may become sticky if you are not properly hydrated, arranging themselves in a pattern called the *rouleaux formation*. This simply means that the blood cells become stuck together and form rows or stacks, making it more difficult for the blood to flow freely through the coronary arteries. Although rouleaux formation is a serious condition, raising the risk of heart attack, it is also reversible with increased water consumption. Alkaline ionized water, of course, is well-suited to this purpose, since its molecular structure and electrical charge enables it to quickly penetrate your cells and hydrate them.

There is a fascinating medical case that demonstrates the healing capacity of alkaline ionized water for cardiovascular disease. According to Dr. Kuwata Keijiroo, a Japanese physician, a thirty-five year old patient suffering from vascular heart disease underwent various treatments over a five-year period, frequently in and out of the hospital. He even endured a major surgical operation. Still, the disease continued to relapse with increasing severity.

Just when the patient began to worry that he would not live much longer, one of his family members heard about ionized water and purchased an ionizer. The patient began to drink alkaline ionized water regularly, and remarkably, his illness responded well. This case history is a compelling one, and it demonstrates the capacity of alkaline ionized water to help treat one of the most deadly chronic degenerative diseases—even when conventional medical interventions cannot.

CONSTIPATION

Constipation, which is medically defined as three or fewer bowel movements per week, is one of the most common health conditions in the United States as well as many other industrialized nations. While it's a well-known fact that most cases of constipation, both temporary and acute, stem mainly from poor diet, inadequate hydration is a much overlooked cause.

Water plays a vital role in the related processes of digestion, metabolism, and elimination of waste material. When there's a low level of H_2O in the gastrointestinal (GI) tract, the breakdown of food into its component parts—nutrients and waste products—is made difficult. A lack of water in the GI tract also means that nutrients cannot be effectively transported to the rest of the body or eliminated via the large intestine. An inadequate supply of water also affects the functioning of organs involved in the digestive process as a whole, including the intestines, kidneys, and liver. As dehydration takes hold in the rest of the body, available water is diverted away from the GI tract to satisfy more pressing needs, making the elimination of solid wastes even more difficult. This is a leading cause of constipation, and the reason why many physicians, myself included, advise chronically constipated patients to drink more water.

Alkaline ionized water can relieve constipation more effectively than other kinds of water due to its unmatched capacity to fully hydrate the body and easily access cells, tissues, and organs. This was shown in a study conducted at Korea's National University School of Medicine by the late Dr. Mu Shik Jhon and Dr. Gyu Hwan Choi. In the study, patients experiencing constipation were instructed to drink alkaline ionized water each day. Within four weeks, approximately 75 percent of the test group enhanced the regularity and frequency of their bowel movements. The study also confirmed that the movement of waste matter through the colon improved by 40 to 60 percent. In my experience, few—if any—products for constipation relief show such dramatic results in so short a time.

EDEMA

The swelling caused by fluid retention in the body's tissues is called *edema*, a disorder also characterized by an excess of salt in the body. Edema, which most commonly affects the legs, ankles, and feet, usually stems from a combination of toxins and the lack of water needed to flush them out of your system. In its water-deprived state, the body shifts into survival mode and begins to hold onto H_2O as well as salt—the substance that allows cells to retain the water they need for proper functioning. As you might expect, a surplus of salt can produce a number of potentially dangerous health problems, beginning with high blood pressure, which is usually the starting point for cardiovascular disease. People who suffer from edema typically have trouble losing weight, exhibit puffiness in their skin, and experience salt cravings triggered by the body's attempt to keep water stores in check.

The conventional treatment for edema is diuretic drugs, which stimulate urination in order to rid the body of toxins. Such treatment is ultimately counterproductive, though, since it creates an even larger water deficit. Cells become more damaged due to lack of water, which is potentially disastrous for the body—particularly when DNA is involved. Additionally, diuretics can have harmful side effects that include cramps, diarrhea, dizziness, increased sensitivity to light, muscle and joint pain, skin rashes, vomiting, and general weakness. In some cases, diuretic use has caused arrhythmia (irregular heartbeat), loss of libido, and impotence. For these reasons, I rarely recommend diuretic drugs as a first course of action for patients with edema. Instead, I address the underlying cause of their condition and focus on rehydrating the body.

Like Dr. Batmanghelidj, who reported that his "water cure" was able to reverse edema in many of his patients, I have found in my own clinical practice that increasing water consumption each day is an effective edema treatment method, provided that patients also follow a healthy diet abundant in potassium-rich vegetables. As daily water intake increases, there is a corresponding increase in urine production, thereby allowing the body to release the salt and toxins it has been storing. Initially, this causes a rise in the frequency of urination, but the body soon adjusts to greater water intake so that the continual need to urinate subsides.

Alkaline ionized water has become my go-to treatment for edema patients (along with a well-balanced diet) because I've found that it solves the problem far more readily than other kinds of H$_2$O. Although ionized water does not eliminate the temporary need to urinate frequently, I've observed its ability to alleviate edema more quickly and easily due to its superior absorbability. Alkaline ionized water hydrates the cells efficiently, allowing them to flush out salt and toxins. I've also noticed that ionized water diminishes skin puffiness and swelling more swiftly, in addition to aiding the weight-loss process.

FATIGUE

Perhaps due to the increasingly busy schedules and longer work hours that characterize our modern world, physicians are reporting that more of their patients complain of fatigue, or lack of energy. Once again, alkaline ionized water offers a simple and highly effective solution to this problem. In order to fully understand why this is the case, you should first be familiar with how the body produces and maintains its energy supply.

Every single cell in your body contains energy factories known as *mitochondria*. These powerhouses are fueled by a substance known as *adenosine triphosphate*, or ATP, which stores energy from the nutrients you take in every day. Proper water intake ensures that your cells will have the nutrients needed to manufacture ATP, since water, which makes up 90 percent of the blood, is the main carrier of vital substances. In addition, as I've noted previously, water is required in order for nutrients to penetrate cell walls, as well as for waste products to be swept out. If this process is impaired by low water levels, your cells literally become tired due to insufficient nutrients and excess buildup.

There is yet another reason why water is so important for energy production in the body— a reason that may be familiar to you if you've ever seen a hydroelectric dam. As its name suggests, the turbines at this kind of dam are powered by the flow of water to generate electricity. A similar process takes place inside your body: Water flows through cellular membranes, and in doing so, rotates cations, which act as energy "pumps" for the cells. This pumping action can work effectively only when there is an adequate flow of water in and out of cells.

In sum, the body relies on hydroelectricity for energy, which is why it's so important to stay well-hydrated. To maximize your body's creation of hydroelectricity, it's best to drink alkaline ionized water, as its distinct hexagonal structure enables it to move quickly through the body, thereby generating more energy. Furthermore, because of the rapid rate at which it travels, ionized H_2O can easily and efficiently provide an energy boost for whatever area of the body is running low. People who regularly drink alkaline ionized water overwhelmingly report greater energy and vitality soon after incorporating it into their lifestyle.

HIGH CHOLESTEROL

According to the American Heart Association, an estimated 102 million adults in the United States have high cholesterol, a condition that has, for decades, been associated with increased risk for heart attack and other forms of heart disease. This link has become widely accepted because of the support it has received from the pharmaceutical industry. Cholesterol-lowering medications, after all, make up a significant portion of the drug industry's total revenue. In recent years, however, more physicians have started to recognize that cholesterol in and of itself is not the problem. What's far more concerning is cholesterol that becomes *oxidized*, a process similar to rusting in which unstable free radicals attack healthy cells. Obviously, the higher your cholesterol levels are, the greater the risk of heart disease becomes once oxidation begins to take place. But this does not mean that cholesterol itself should be feared.

In actuality, cholesterol is a necessary, natural substance. It's found in every human body, whether young or old, active or inactive, thin or overweight, healthy or unhealthy. Cholesterol is needed to maintain cell walls and produce many hormones as well as vitamin D, a nutrient that acts as a hormone, and one in which many people are deficient. Cholesterol is also found in a variety of foods, particularly meat and dairy products. Although some of the foods in these categories promote a well-balanced diet when consumed in moderation, most of them, particularly when eaten in large quantities, raise the level of unhealthy cholesterol in your system. As a result, doctors recommend that these foods be avoided, especially by those who are at high risk for heart disease or have already developed various cardiovascular disorders. I agree with this recommendation, but not for the same reason.

The primary danger involved in eating foods like beef, cheese, and eggs is not their high cholesterol content, but their acidifying effects. Because they create an acidic internal environment, a diet consisting of such foods will lead to chronic inflammation and free radical damage, both of which dramatically increase the risk of heart disease. Thus, rather than concentrate on regulating cholesterol levels per se, I advise patients to follow a diet that supports acid-alkaline balance to prevent oxidation and inflammation.

Furthermore, as Dr. Batmanghelidj discovered decades ago, there is a direct correlation between high cholesterol and body dehydration. In fact, his research has conclusively shown that dehydration—not diet—is the chief cause of cholesterol buildup in the heart's tissues and arteries. When cells face the threat of inadequate water supply, cholesterol deposits collect around cellular walls in an effort to retain H_2O. The longer the dehydrated state persists, the greater the cellular cholesterol buildup.

Compounding this problem is the fact that the blood becomes thicker when the body's water supply is low, as H_2O is required to facilitate the digestive process and break down food into microscopic particles. This poses a serious health hazard, since blood thickening increases the risk of stroke, heart attack, and other heart-related conditions, especially when the blood is also acidic. Blood that is thicker *and* acidic encourages the production of cholesterol and causes damage to arterial walls, creating small tears and abrasions in its lining. When this occurs, the body is forced to produce even more cholesterol to form a protective covering over the corroded walls. This "vulnerable plaque," as it is called, is extremely fragile and susceptible to rupture, which is why it is one of the leading causes of heart attack and stroke. In sum, dehydration and over-acidity combine to create a truly vicious cycle in which the body is forced to produce ever-increasing levels of cholesterol to cope with its low water supply and thick acidic blood.

However, when the body is properly hydrated, cholesterol levels are kept in check and, as Dr. Batmanghelidj found, also reduced. Drinking alkaline ionized water is a better means to this end because of how quickly it is transported and absorbed in the body, as well as its high pH value, which helps to restore acid-alkaline balance and reverse inflammation. Moreover, alkaline ionized water lessens the thickness of the blood, driving down cholesterol levels in the bloodstream. When it comes to high cholesterol, you can literally drink your problems away with alkaline ionized water.

HYPERTENSION

The Centers for Disease Control and Prevention estimate that one out of three adults is afflicted with *hypertension,* or high blood pressure, and that an additional 25 percent has prehypertension, meaning they are at heightened risk. These statistics highlight the need for major lifestyle change, particularly in terms of diet. As Dr. Kancho Kinanaka, a pioneer of ionized water treatment, has asserted, people with high blood pressure also suffer from acidosis "virtually without exception." He has observed many cases in which alkaline ionized water successfully lowered blood pressure, and he offers several explanations for this.

First, because the water improves oxygenation of the body, the heart does not have to work as hard to pump blood. As you may recall from Chapter 4, a sufficient amount of oxygen is required for the heart to function efficiently, and alkaline ionized water fulfills this need. Second, the high pH value of the water decreases the blood thickening that occurs when the body is acidified, dehydrated, and in a hypertensive state, thereby lowering blood pressure. Finally, alkaline ionized water is rich in calcium ions, which help dissolve plaque and cholesterol buildup in the arterial walls, reopening the passageways for quicker and more efficient blood transport. For these reasons, alkaline ionized water is an ideal remedy for hypertension.

PREMATURE AGING

Premature aging, a term used to describe aging that occurs at an accelerated pace, is characterized by declining function of the body's organ systems. Physicians measure premature aging by comparing *chronological age,* the actual age of an individual, to their *biological age,* which is based on the condition of organs and overall function of the body. Biological age can be found by evaluating the patient's physiological functioning against that of an average healthy person during each decade of life. Ideally, chronological and biological age should be the same; however, it is not uncommon today for adults to have a biological age equivalent to a person five, ten, and even twenty years older—a sure sign of premature aging.

The significant rise in the prevalence of this condition in recent years is most commonly attributed to factors such as a diet high in fat and sugar, lack of exercise, environmental pollution, and stress. But the causes that remain mostly ignored are bodily dehydration and acid-alkaline imbalance.

Dehydration

The theory that water loss—specifically, the loss of hexagonal H_2O—is the primary cause of premature aging is supported by two basic facts of human physiology that have long been recognized and studied by scientists:

1. **The amount of water in the human body declines with age.** In fact, this decline begins almost immediately after birth, at which time the body is more than 90 percent water. By the time an infant is one year of age, water constitutes only 70 percent of the body and levels off until old age—the bodies of older adults are typically 50 percent water or less. Therefore, it's no wonder that so many other debilitating health conditions also arise in old age.

2. **The speed at which water flows in and out of cells, tissues, and organs decreases with age.** Speed of water flow is important, since it can affect the amount of water in the cell's internal environment in relation to its external environment. When the flow of water slows down as you age, the amount inside cells is reduced from an optimal 60 percent to as low as 40 percent. Obviously, the consequences for cellular function are countless.

Based on these two facts, it's easy to see why proper hydration is so important to maintain, especially as you get older. But as you're well aware by now, the *quality* of the water you drink is just (if not more) important as the quantity. It isn't enough to drink eight 8-ounce glasses of water daily; you should also drink water that is the most easily transported, distributed, and absorbed. The structural and chemical composition of ionized water makes it uniquely suited to this purpose. Its hexagonal shape, small cluster size, and low surface tension allow the water to reach all of your body's cells and fully hydrate each one. Your tissues and organs will never be at a loss for H_2O, which is crucial for slowing down the aging process and boosting vitality.

Acid-Alkaline Imbalance

As Chapter 2 explains, acid-alkaline imbalance is a growing health concern in the modern world, and over-acidity, or acidosis, is the more commonly occurring problem—particularly in Western societies like the United States, where diets are high in acidifying foods. Blood acidity is difficult to reverse with food alone, so even when you increase your intake of alkalizing foods, the imbalance can persist. Acidic waste products continue to accumulate in cells, tissues, and organs, altering their structure and impeding proper function. In fact, the root cause of premature aging is the loss of cellular integrity, since it sets the stage for the development of disease and other unhealthy conditions.

Alkaline ionized water rectifies this situation by neutralizing acidity and discharging wastes from cells, all while hydrating the body. The water is tailor-made for this purpose with its high alkaline pH and natural absorbability. As it hydrates the body, ionized H_2O simultaneously flushes out toxins and waste products, maintains proper flow of water in and out of cells, and hinders the buildup of acids. By supporting the proper function of cells, tissues, and organs, your entire body is fortified against premature aging. To quote Sang Whang, a renowned Korean scientist and author of *Reverse Aging*, "I have . . . seen [people] who have gotten healthier and younger looking without diet or exercises, by simply drinking alkaline [ionized] water."

TYPE 2 DIABETES

Type 2 diabetes, also known as adult-onset diabetes, occurs when the body is no longer able to produce enough of the hormone *insulin* or when your cells are unable to respond to it. Insulin is needed for the transportation of glucose, one of the body's chief sources of energy, from the blood to the cells so that it can be used for fueling the body. When you are insulin resistant, the movement of glucose does not occur, overloading the blood with insulin and depriving the cells of required energy. The consequences of this hormonal dysfunction can be fatal if left untreated.

Doctors have identified several risk factors for type 2 diabetes, including high blood pressure, a high-fat diet, and a sedentary lifestyle. There is also a genetic component in the development of type 2 diabetes, and some groups are at higher risk than others. For instance, larger numbers of African Americans, Native Americans, Hispanics, and the elderly suffer from the disease. Yet, water deficiency, a prime factor affecting the body's energy levels and regulation of glucose, is rarely discussed as an indirect cause of diabetes. As Dr. Batmanghelidj discovered decades ago, the development of type 2 diabetes is closely tied to a low supply of water in the brain, which utilizes glucose instead of H_2O for energy during periods of dehydration. In order to maintain normal function, the brain summons increased amounts of glucose, causing sugar content in the blood to rise significantly. High blood sugar levels force the body to produce more and more insulin, and when it can no longer keep up with blood glucose levels, diabetes develops.

Another way dehydration is related to type 2 diabetes involves the genes. As I mentioned, most doctors and scientists today acknowledge that a strong link exists between type 2 diabetes and genetics. Your genetic information is contained in DNA, whose day-to-day functions include manufacturing proteins and other materials needed for cellular function. DNA can perform these activities only if the body is sufficiently hydrated, since water is needed in order for DNA strands to maintain their structure. A low water supply increases the probability of DNA-coding errors, which may result in a genetic mutation or abnormality. Hence, water is absolutely crucial when it comes to genetic coding, something that is strongly correlated with type 2 diabetes.

Dr. Batmanghelidj, who treated a number of diabetes patients during his lifetime, argued that water and salt, which regulates water levels in the body, "will reverse adult-onset diabetes in its early stages. Not recognizing adult-onset diabetes as a complication of dehydration will, in time, cause massive damage to the blood vessels all over the body." By advising his patients to increase their daily water intake, Dr. Batmanghelidj was successful in his efforts to improve several cases of type 2 diabetes, even reversing the condition in many patients. However, it was Dr. Kuwata Keijiroo of Japan who first tested and observed the greater effectiveness of alkaline ionized water in the treatment of diabetics. According to Dr. Keijiroo, the patients who consumed the alkaline and antioxidant-rich H_2O for only one month experienced significant reductions in blood and urine glucose levels. In fact, sugar in the urine was found to completely disappear, with minimal glucose concentration remaining in the blood.

Another study published in a 2007 issue of the *Biological and Pharmaceutical Bulletin* supported Dr. Keijiroo's results. A group of researchers tested the effects of alkaline ionized water on diabetic mice, and ultimately found that it reduced glucose concentration, increased blood insulin levels, improved glucose tolerance, and preserved pancreatic cells, which are responsible for insulin secretion. Based on their study, the scientists concluded that alkaline ionized water would also benefit humans with type 2 diabetes. Unfortunately, ionized H_2O is most likely not an effective treatment for type 1 diabetes, an autoimmune disorder with no known exact cause. Healthy drinking water is still important for type 1 diabetics, but there is no medical evidence that suggests the benefits of alkaline ionized water would have an impact on the disease.

CONCLUSION

Alkaline ionized water is tremendously beneficial for your health, and the medical conditions it can be used to treat are not limited to the ones discussed in this chapter. Drinking alkaline H_2O has proven effective in cases of more specific ailments such as hay fever, osteoporosis, and various skin problems, including eczema. (See Chapter 6 for more about ionized water and skin care.) It can also alleviate the common discomforts associated with digestive disorders like diarrhea, flatulence (bloating), indigestion, and nausea. As you read this, scientists are in the process of researching other ways that alkaline ionized water can be used medicinally. I am confident they will soon identify other conditions that can be greatly improved, if not completely eliminated, by drinking water that is pure, hydrating, alkaline, and rich in minerals and antioxidants.

As with any health-boosting product or endeavor, the quickness with which results are seen may vary according to individual medical issues and levels of overall health. Most often, the people who notice differences in the shortest amount of time are those who begin a regimen of alkaline ionized water when they are ill or experiencing specific symptoms. On other hand, I have had healthy patients tell me that they observed positive changes after only a week of drinking ionized water.

There's simply no way to accurately predict how alkaline ionized H_2O will affect every person, no matter how many times I'm asked to do so. What I can say with certainty is that anyone who drinks this water on a daily basis will see definite improvements in their health that will become more noticeable over time. For most people, a water pH of 8 to 8.5 should be sufficient, but you should slowly increase the amount you drink each day. (See Chapter 8 for more about ionized water regimens.) If you consume this water safely and regularly, you will literally be drinking to and for your health.

6

The Health Benefits of Acidic Ionized Water

Water is the world's most vital resource, but it's also one of the most wasted. Water filtration systems such as reverse osmosis (RO) filters aren't just ineffective—they're uneconomical and environmentally unfriendly. For every gallon of water produced by an RO filter, one gallon is also wasted. Water ionizers, an asset to your health *and* the environment, are the complete opposite. Although the term "acidic" is usually assumed to be negative, acidic ionized water has properties that favor your well-being. Moreover, acidic H_2O is multifunctional, with everyday applications that range from skin care to food sanitation. As you consume alkaline water for internal wellness, you can put the other ionized byproduct to practical use as a sterilizing agent, powerful disinfectant, and hygiene product for your skin, hair, and teeth. By ionizing your water, you ensure that nothing goes to waste, and you rejuvenate your whole self—inside and out.

It's important to remember that acidic ionized water is for topical use *only* and should not be taken internally. Made up primarily of hydrogen ions, the water is oxidizing and therefore can cause extensive free radical damage. It also goes without saying that the water is very acidifying, so it can wreak havoc on your system's acid-alkaline balance. Still, when used for external purposes, acidic ionized water acts as a protective shield against harmful bacteria that can cause unsightly skin conditions and serious medical problems like heart disease. In addition, washing your food with acidic ionized water is a useful preventive action against food poisoning and contamination. This chapter focuses on the various health issues for which acidic ionized water offers effective relief and treatment.

DENTAL AND ORAL BACTERIA

Whether due to diabetes, genetics, hormonal changes, stress, or deficient hygiene, dental plaque and tartar is a common problem. *Plaque* forms when bacteria in the mouth combine with mucus, creating a sticky white substance that adheres to the surface of the teeth. *Tartar* is plaque that becomes hardened, and it is nearly impossible to remove with a regular toothbrush. Left untreated, the accumulation of plaque and tartar can lead to *gingivitis,* or gum inflammation, which eventually develops into periodontal (gum) disease.

More alarmingly, the bacteria that compose plaque and tartar can break away from your teeth and travel deeper into the body, ultimately reaching your bloodstream. To protect itself, the body produces more cholesterol; but, in excess, this substance can cause narrowing of the arteries and other problems that may result in heart disease. For this reason, many doctors today are taking an interest in their patients' teeth and gums, stressing proper dental hygiene and recommending regular visits to the dentist.

Because of its antibacterial properties, acidic ionized water nicely complements regular dental and oral hygiene habits. Brushing your teeth with it will help to keep your teeth free of plaque and tartar, and using the water as a mouthwash will wipe out any bacteria lingering on your gums and tongue, as well as relieve mouth sores and sore throats. Just be sure to spit the water out when you're finished, as swallowing acidic water will upset your internal balance.

FOOD POISONING

In the last several years, there has been an alarming rise in the incidence of food contamination, forcing product recalls and inciting outbreaks of food poisoning. The chief culprits are *Escherichia coli,* more widely known as *E. coli,* and salmonella, both of which are primarily foodborne bacteria that, when ingested, can cause severe infections in the gastrointestinal and urinary tracts. Several cases of food contamination due to *E. coli* and salmonella have been documented since the 1960s. The bacteria has tainted a wide range of foods, including meat and dairy products, poultry, spinach, cantaloupe, and peanuts.

There are many reasons for the relatively recent surge in food safety issues. First of all, most of the foods sold in supermarkets are now shipped all over the country or imported from overseas before finally arriving on local store shelves. This provides plenty of opportunity for bacteria to breed and grow. Compounding this problem is the fact that much of the nation's food supply—about 95 percent—is not adequately inspected, if inspected at all. The Food and Drug Administration (FDA) and United States Department of Agriculture (USDA) lack the necessary resources and manpower, and the commercial interests that oversee the food industry have made the process more difficult.

Clearly, we cannot rely on the government alone to safeguard our health. It's up to each of us to make smart choices when buying and preparing food. I recommend choosing organic foods that are locally grown whenever possible, as well as buying meat and dairy that comes from free-range and grass-fed animals, and fish that are wild-caught. It's equally important to take precautions when handling and cleaning food—and this is where acidic ionized water can play an indispensable role. Based on several studies conducted in the United States since 1999, scientists have determined that acidic ionized H_2O is an effective form of food sanitation and protection.

Some studies focused solely on the water's antimicrobial effects on the food itself. In 2002, a research team at Pennsylvania State University compared the ability of acidic ionized water (with a pH of about 2.6) to reduce the amount of salmonella in contaminated poultry against standard sanitizing methods. They submerged carcasses in different substances, and ultimately found that the acidic ionized water was equally effective as the other chemical compounds, which included acetic acid and trisodium phosphate. However, the researchers concluded that acidic water was the superior method, sharing neither the cost nor the adverse environmental effects of the other sterilizing agents. The acidic water was later studied by the university's Department of Agricultural and Biological Engineering in 2003, which, using alfalfa seeds and sprouts, tested its effectiveness in killing a strain of *E. coli*. They measured the reduction of *E. coli* over intervals of 2, 4, 8, 16, 32, and 64 minutes, finding that the E. coli was decreased by as much as 97.1 percent in the treated seeds and 99.8 percent in the sprouts. The longer they were soaked in the acidic ionized water, the greater the reduction of *E. coli* in the sprouts and seeds, which were not at all damaged by acidic water exposure. Since then, research has shown that the water can significantly reduce and eradicate harmful bacteria and fungi—including *E. coli* and salmonella—in cucumbers, eggs, lettuce, poultry, seafood, strawberries, and tomatoes, as well as many meat products.

Scientists at the University of Connecticut have also examined the effects of acidic ionized water on the bacteria present on cooking implements—an important factor to consider when preparing food. They exposed plastic cutting boards to culture strains of *E. coli* and listeria, a harmful bacterium also known to cause food poisoning. The cutting boards were divided into two groups. Half were soaked in acidic ionized water, and the other half in sterilized non-ionized water. The acidic H_2O successfully wiped out the bacteria on the cutting boards, whereas the pathogens submerged in the non-ionized water survived. A comparable study found that acidic ionized water is also an effective method for deactivating a variety of bacteria on surfaces such as glass, ceramic tile (glazed and unglazed), and vitreous china.

HAIR DAMAGE

Like your skin, healthy hair is slightly acidic, having an average pH of 5.6. And, like many skin-care products and cosmetics, various shampoos and conditioners can disrupt your hair's normal pH level, causing dryness, split ends, and other mild hair damage. By rinsing your hair with acidic ionized water after a shower, you will not only clean it thoroughly, but also maintain its natural luster. Topical use of the water may also reverse conditions of the scalp, including dandruff and psoriasis. Regularly drinking alkaline ionized water and following a healthy alkalizing diet will help to reduce internal over-acidity that may be causing hair and scalp problems. It's also important that you buy hair products that boost, not hinder, pH balance.

SKIN AGING

Here's a fascinating fact about your skin: A single square inch contains three million cells, each one of which is replaced every thirty days. In healthy people, these regenerated skin cells are equally healthy and vibrant. But this does not occur in most adults, and the tendency towards dull skin only increases with age. In fact, it's often considered to be a natural consequence of the aging process. This, however, is not the case. Truly healthy people continue to have good skin throughout their lives, and one reason is acid-alkaline balance, along with proper nutrition and other lifestyle factors.

Internal balance has a significant effect on your skin, since regeneration will not occur when the body's inner environment is chronically acidic. But external balance, or the acid-alkaline equilibrium on the surface of your skin, is just as important. Unlike your body's internal environment, which thrives in a slightly alkaline state, the ideal pH for your skin is between 5.4 and 5.9. When it falls outside this slightly acidic range for a prolonged period, skin tone may begin to wane, and many of the facial cleansers and cosmetic products marketed as solutions to this problem further disrupt the skin's normal pH levels rather than balance them. This is because many soaps and refining agents, including makeup, have a higher pH than the skin, thereby depleting its natural acids and making it more difficult to neutralize harmful microbes. Even when these products are rinsed off, they leave behind residue that can clog pores and diminish your skin's ability to guard against bacteria by causing dryness, flakiness, and wrinkles. The ultimate result is skin that ages more rapidly.

Topical application of acidic ionized water can put a stop to skin aging and vastly improve the condition of your skin if it has already started to lose its healthful glow. The acidifying effect of the water helps to restore normal pH to the skin's surface, thus reviving its antimicrobial properties. This will allow your skin to retain a youthful appearance as well as keep it soft and supple. Acidic ionized water also acts as a natural astringent, which means that it tightens the skin and prevents the formation of wrinkles. For this reason, the water can serve as an excellent substitute for aftershave lotions, producing smoother and cleaner shaves.

SKIN CONDITIONS

Your skin is an important part of your immune system, acting as a protective barrier against microorganisms that are attempting to penetrate deeper into your body. The skin is also an organ of elimination, ridding the body of toxins through perspiration. However, the successful execution of these functions may come at the cost of skin health, particularly when proper internal and external pH levels are not maintained. If the body is too acidic internally and too alkaline externally, toxins—both those trying to infect the body and those being forced out—build up and clog pores, leading to blemishes, blotchiness, excessively oily skin, and poor skin tone. For people who are predisposed to skin problems, embarrassing and painful conditions such as acne, eczema, psoriasis, and shingles can develop. These conditions are made worse by skin-care products and medications that diminish the acidity of the skin's surface, in effect weakening its ability to fight bacteria and infection. Thus, a vicious cycle emerges.

Acidic ionized water, especially when used in combination with its alkaline counterpart, is an extremely potent remedy for skin disorders. Its low pH returns the skin to a slightly acidic state, which reactivates its ability to kill microorganisms like *propionibacterium acnes*—an acne-causing bacterium. Additionally, its small cluster size allows it to sink deeply into pores, destroying the bacteria that lurk beneath the skin's surface. When paired with a regimen of alkaline ionized water (as well as a diet of alkalizing foods), acidic ionized water creates an environment where harmful bacteria can no longer thrive, preventing skin conditions or hastening their reversal.

I have witnessed a dramatic example of such a turnaround. When my daughter was seven years old, she developed *eczema*, a disorder in which the skin becomes irritated and inflamed, causing itchy rashes, painful blisters, and peeling. By the time she was seventeen, the eczema patches on her arms were dark red in color and would often ooze. Embarrassed, she made sure to wear shirts that covered her arms, even in the middle of the summer. Every healing modality we tried was ineffective, which was enough to convince us that she would suffer from the condition for the rest of her life—that is, until I learned about the benefits of ionized water. I immediately purchased an ionizer for my home, had my daughter drink plenty of alkaline ionized water throughout the day, and applied the acidic water to her arms a few times daily. After only four days, the eczema completely disappeared, and the scarring it had caused faded significantly.

Similarly, acidic ionized water has been shown to accelerate the healing of *shingles*, a painful condition caused by the herpes zoster virus also responsible for chickenpox. Shingles most often occurs when the dormant chickenpox virus is reactivated at some point in adulthood to produce a painful, blistering, and bumpy rash. These blisters fill with pus, erupt to form scabs, and often leave unattractive scars. Most doctors recommend applying cool compresses to the rashes to soothe and dry out the blisters, and then washing the affected areas with mild soap and water several times a day. Using acidic ionized water for this same purpose speeds up the recovery process because it provides relief, disinfects the area, *and* kills the root of the problem—the virus. The acidic ionized H_2O also minimizes scarring, as in the case of my daughter's eczema.

For optimal results, apply acidic ionized water to your face and neck twice a day—once in the morning and once before you go to bed. You can even add one or two gallons of acidic water to your tub when taking a bath. Coupled with an alkaline water regimen, you will notice definite improvements in your complexion. However, it's important to keep in mind that additional medication may be necessary to reduce inflammation and relieve the pain that accompanies skin conditions like the ones mentioned above. You should always consult your health-care provider or dermatologist if you experience symptoms that persist without improvement.

SKIN INFECTIONS AND WOUNDS

Because acidic ionized water neutralizes bacteria and viruses that attack the body, it functions as a powerful sterilizing agent. Many doctors in other countries have used the substance as an antiseptic for over a decade, applying it to minor scrapes and cuts as well as more serious infections such as bedsores and *methicillin-resistant Staphylococcus aureus* (MRSA), which are growing concerns in hospitals throughout the world. In addition, the water has been found to speed up the healing process for skin wounds and infections, giving it a twofold treatment function.

The effectiveness of acidic ionized water as a wound disinfectant and healer has been documented in a number of studies. One of these was conducted by researchers at Russia's Moscow State University in 2004 and was specifically designed to investigate the antibacterial actions of the acidic ionized water on ten of the most common hospital infections. Most of these infectious agents were completely deactivated within thirty seconds of being inoculated with the water; the others were killed within five minutes. Another 2004 experiment, this time administered by Japanese scientists, tested the effects of various types of electrolyzed (ionized) water on skin wounds, using rats as subjects. The scientists found that acidic ionized water was most effective for accelerating the healing process, leading them to the theory that the water furthered the growth of *fibroblasts*, specialized cells involved in skin regeneration. In other words, acidic ionized water not only disinfects wounds and protects them from infection, but also improves the body's ability to grow new, healthy skin.

The antiseptic and therapeutic effects of acidic ionized water have resulted in new treatment methods that are now commonly practiced in many Japanese and Russian hospitals. Doctors have reported dramatic improvements in disease complications like diabetic ulcers, which are extremely dangerous when they become infected and occasionally require amputation. Ionized water has proven to be a major medical breakthrough for this condition, and Japanese physicians have successfully treated several cases of diabetic ulcer using a combination of acidic and alkaline H_2O. The acidic component, which is given a very low pH of about 2.5, is applied topically several times a day while the alkaline water, with a pH of 8 to 10, is consumed in place of regular tap water. This twofold method has controlled infection, reversed gangrene, and saved entire limbs from being amputated.

The incredible success rate of ionized water treatment is captured in a Japanese documentary entitled *Miracle Water* that aired on the national public television station in 1996. The documentary, which was made at the urging of the government's Ministry of Health, chronicles the treatment and rehabilitation of a diabetic patient named Mr. Abe (pronounced *Ah-bay*), who is dangerously close to having his gangrenous foot and toe amputated when the film begins. He opts to undergo ionized water treatment, drinking alkaline water and bathing his ulcers in the acidic water several times a day. Over the course of the documentary, viewers can clearly see his feet and toes steadily improving, and ultimately, Mr. Abe is released from the hospital without having to endure amputation or surgery.

Topical solutions of acidic ionized water have also been used effectively to manage liver abscesses and treat MRSA, a dangerous "super bug" that can develop as a post-operative infection and is difficult to treat with antibiotics. According to the researchers who tested its effects, acid ionized water significantly reduced the occurrence of post-surgical infections in patients, particularly those who underwent open heart surgery.

Because of its effectiveness in eliminating and healing wounds and infections, acidic ionized water has several applications in a medical setting. Doctors can use the water to sterilize instruments from endoscopes to dialysis machines and to disinfect hospital tap water. But the functionality of the water goes beyond the doctor's office and hospital. It may be employed by athletes to get rid of rashes like "jock's itch" or fungal infections such as athlete's foot. Others may apply it to bug bites, stings, and skin irritations like poison ivy and poison oak to relieve itchiness. However you use the water, you will be ensuring your protection against potentially harmful bacteria and speeding up your body's healing process.

ACIDIC IONIZED WATER pH RANGES AND THEIR USES	
Water pH Range	**Uses**
5.5 to 6.5	• Brushing teeth
	• Improving complexion and skin tone
	• Rinsing mouth and hair
	• Storing produce to maintain freshness
5.5 to 4.5	• Cleaning glass surfaces
	• Healing burns, cuts, and minor scrapes
	• Improving complexion and skin tone
	• Neutralizing foot odor and fungal infections
	• Soaking produce to kill bacteria
	• Sterilizing cooking implements such as cutting boards
	• Tightening the skin
	• Treating pimples, mild rashes, and skin tags
4.5 to 3.5	• Healing and preventing infection of skin wounds
	• Relieving itchiness
	• Treating insect bites, stings, and rashes due to poison ivy or oak
	• Treating skin conditions such as acne, eczema, and psoriasis, and less serious infections like athlete's foot
3.5 to 2.5*	• Destroying pathogens in contaminated food
	• Treating severe skin conditions and wounds, such as diabetic ulcers, gangrene, and MRSA

Not all water ionizers allow settings as low as 2.5.

USING ACIDIC IONIZED WATER

Since acidic ionized water has a wide range of functions, it may be necessary to adjust the pH setting on your water ionizer. The table on page 76 categorizes the various uses of acidic ionized water discussed in this chapter according to the appropriate pH range. As you can see from the table, the lowest pH levels are reserved for more extreme cases, and even then should be administered by a professional. For most purposes, a pH of 4 to 6 should be sufficient.

Keep in mind that you should not attempt to treat a serious condition with acidic ionized water unless instructed or supervised by a physician. Start with a pH level that is lowest in acidity and, if you do not see results, gradually increase its strength. For more tips for using your water ionizer, see Chapter 8.

CONCLUSION

Although its use requires a bit more caution, acidic ionized water can be just as beneficial to your health as its alkaline counterpart. The substance has everyday applications that can transform your life, from your hygiene to the safety of your food to the cleanliness of your kitchen. You can even guarantee lasting freshness of plants and flowers, as acidic ionized H_2O also acts as a plant stimulant. The functionality and health-giving properties of acidic ionized water provide one more reason why water ionizers are an economical solution to wasteful water filtration, and why having one in your home can be so advantageous. (See Chapter 8 for more on buying and using a water ionizer.) You can cleanse your body *and* environment, any day, any time. When used together, acidic and alkaline water promote a holistic approach to health.

However, to maximize the benefits of ionized water, you need to take care of your health in other ways, and you can start with your diet. As I've mentioned throughout this book, the foods you eat have a major impact on your internal environment and can easily disturb your acid-alkaline balance. By following the nutritional guidelines outlined in the next chapter, you will reinforce the positive effects of ionized water and further enhance your overall wellness.

7

Eating and Drinking for Acid-Alkaline Balance

Throughout this book, I have stressed the central role that acid-alkaline balance plays in your health, which is one of the many reasons why water ionizers are such worthwhile investments. The alkaline water relieves internal toxic burdens caused by over-acidity, while the acidic water restores pH balance to your skin and hair, thereby preventing infection and further damage. However, ionized water will not alone enable you to attain ideal wellness. You also need to make dietary choices that reinforce the powerful healing effects of alkaline and acidic H_2O so that your body is perfectly poised to combat disease. Therefore, it's important that you follow certain nutritional guidelines that support acid-alkaline balance—something you can do only if you're aware of the various acidifying, alkalizing, and neutral effects produced by the foods and beverages you consume. The following pages provide an overview of the relationship between your diet and pH balance as well as the information necessary to make smarter choices when eating and drinking for your health.

BASIC NUTRITIONAL GUIDELINES FOR ACHIEVING pH BALANCE

Although the nutritional content of food tends to be emphasized more than its impact on pH, everything you eat and drink leaves its imprint on the body in the form of acidifying or alkalizing residue. After foods are digested and metabolized, they produce food ash that generally raises or lowers pH levels depending on the type of food and its mineral content. How a certain food interacts with your internal environment in this way is actually more important than the food's inherent pH value—the level of acidity or alkalinity prior to consumption. Not all foods that are inherently acidic will be acidifying, nor will every inherently alkaline food have an alkalizing effect when metabolized. For example, acidic foods like citrus fruits actually alkalize the body after being digested. Therefore, knowing the effect a particular food or beverage will have on your pH level is the key to selecting them wisely. It's also the key to optimal nutrition, since acid-alkaline imbalance interrupts the proper absorption and utilization of nutrients, which may result in a nutritional deficiency.

In general, alkalizing foods should comprise 60 to 80 percent of your daily diet. If your pH level is slightly acidic, closer to 80 percent of your intake each day should come from alkalizing sources. Basically, the lower your pH level, the more alkalizing foods and beverages you need to consume. An ideal diet consists of a higher proportion of alkalizing foods at every meal and snack, thereby enabling your body to neutralize the acids produced during digestion as well as reduce acidic buildup. This method is more effective than cramming alkalizing foods into one or two meals and consuming solely acidifying foods for the rest of the day. You should also avoid eating meals and snacks consisting entirely of acidifying foods, such as steak and potatoes or pasta and meatballs. Include an alkalizing food source like green vegetables to add some balance and diminish acidification. The only exception to this rule is the rare case of over-alkalinity, a condition that necessitates increasing consumption of acidifying foods until pH balance is restored.

When you first begin to modify your diet for acid-alkaline balance, you should consume alkalizing foods and drinks in greater amounts. When your pH reaches an optimal level (a slightly alkaline range of 7.365 to 7.45), you can gradually reduce the daily amount of alkalizing foods you eat. Additionally, your diet can be adjusted based on how much alkaline ionized water you drink each day. Once you achieve a balanced and stable pH level, you may even find that you can eat equal amounts of alkalizing and acidifying foods without any problems. Still, I recommend that you continue to eat a higher proportion of alkalizing foods even after you achieve acid-alkaline balance, as they tend to be more nutritionally beneficial.

As you embark on a new diet plan and become more mindful of pH balance, you may consider drastically shrinking your intake of acidifying foods and beverages, or abolishing them from your diet. *Do not do so*—acidifying foods can also be nutritious. Indeed, your body requires foods that are rich in protein—meat, fish, eggs, milk, and dairy products—in order to function properly. More important, your body needs a certain amount of acidifying protein to produce and retain a supply of alkaline minerals, which protect your cells and tissues from harmful acids. When your alkaline mineral reserves are depleted, the body is overcome by acids because it lacks the resources necessary for neutralizing them. The end result is greater acidity, and, therefore, heightened risk of disease.

However, there are scenarios that call for an all-alkaline diet, such as cases of pronounced acidosis, a severe imbalance that may be accompanied by painful symptoms. An entirely alkaline diet of fruits and vegetables allows the body to quickly recover from an overly acidic state. Still, all-alkaline diets should not be followed for more than one to two weeks. As soon as the symptoms begin to subside, it's best to resume a more balanced eating plan. Keep in mind that each person has his or her own unique biochemistry that shapes how certain foods and beverages affect the body. Pay careful attention to how you feel after each meal, and adjust your diet accordingly.

ACIDIFYING AND ALKALIZING FOODS

Now that you're more familiar with the relationship between food and pH balance, it's important that you also know which foods are acidifying, alkalizing, or neutral. Generally speaking, very few foods and beverages are truly *neutral*, both in terms of inherent pH value and effect on the body. Most sources categorize foods and other substances as having low, medium, or high alkalizing and acidifying effects, but even this is not a foolproof classification system. Each food's ranking on the acid-alkaline scale is not always clear-cut. For this reason, the foods discussed in this section are labeled only as "acidifying" or "alkalizing" with the understanding that their effects can range from mild to significant. I have also limited my discussion to only the most common foods, so this listing is not a comprehensive or definitive one. Also, continue to keep in mind that genetic and biochemical factors, as well as food quality, may influence how a certain substance acts in your body. If you find that you have a hypersensitivity to a food, you should probably avoid it altogether—no matter how beneficial it's supposed to be—and compensate for its absence with other foods that can provide the same health-boosting effects.

Acidifying Foods and Beverages

Foods and drinks that produce an acidifying, or acid-forming, effect in the body are generally those that are high in protein, fat, and carbohydrates. This is because proteins and fats are broken down into amino acids and fatty acids, respectively, during the process of digestion. In addition, the basic building block of carbohydrates is glucose, which is poorly converted by the body and therefore produces acid-forming elements. The main acidifying food categories are outlined below.

Alcohol

All alcoholic beverages cause body acidification, so it's not surprising that excessive alcohol consumption is linked to diseases like cirrhosis of the liver. The problem lies in one of its byproducts, *acetaldehyde*, which forms when alcohol is metabolized and converted into a type of acid. When the chemical accumulates, it has significant toxic effects that can lead to liver damage. However, drinking alcohol on occasion will not pose a hazard to your health. On the contrary, recent research indicates that moderate consumption of beer or wine, particularly red wine due to its antioxidant content, can enhance your well-being by relieving stress and improving digestion. I recommend no more than one drink per day for women and no more than two drinks for men. A glass of water should accompany your alcoholic beverage in order to keep acidification to a minimum.

Artificial Sweeteners

Many people seeking to eliminate sugar from their diet replace it with artificial sweeteners under the mistaken but widely held belief that they are healthier. However, sugar substitutes such as aspartame (NutraSweet), saccharin, and cyclamates are extremely acidifying, and many of the chemical ingredients they contain have been connected to a host of disease conditions and symptoms. If you are looking for a sugar substitute, stevia or xylitol are acceptable alternatives. In general, though, it's better to eat naturally occurring sugar in sparing amounts—while avoiding added sugars—than to put chemical sweeteners into your body.

Caffeine Products

The foods and beverages in this group include chocolate, cocoa, tea, and all forms of coffee, including decaffeinated (which is not entirely caffeine-free). Caffeine promotes the production of mucus in the body as well as large amounts of acidic residue. And despite the fact that most people today drink coffee for more energy, the substance actually depletes the body's energy reserves. This creates a vicious cycle in which the coffee drinker seeks another caffeine fix as soon as the initial boost of artificial energy subsides—the cups of coffee add up, but your energy does not. By maintaining acid-alkaline balance, you can avoid this problem and still have all the energy you need—and more.

Condiments (Processed)

Although most commercial food products are undesirable dietary choices, the main culprits in this category are ketchup, mayonnaise, mustard, and soy sauce. Like the vast majority of processed foods, they contain a significant amount of sugar and unnatural additives that have acidifying properties, and thus can throw your pH off kilter. Instead of using condiments to flavor your food, you should consider nutritious and far healthier substitutes such as natural herbs and spices, sea salt, and kelp. If you would rather not eliminate ketchup and mustard completely, use them sparingly and always choose organic brands, which can be found at your local supermarket and health food store.

Grains

Refined and whole grains, a group that includes millet, oats, rice, and wheat, are generally acidifying. This is because grains are primarily composed of carbohydrates, a substance that is often not easily digested—especially when you are unknowingly allergic or sensitive to the grains—and tends to be very acid-forming. In addition, grains contain *phytic acid,* a chemical that both acidifies the body and blocks the absorption of vital nutrients. However, when grains are sprouted, they are alkalizing and positively impact your body in ways similar to green vegetables. In addition, sprouted grains are rich in vitamins, minerals, and other essential nutrients. I strongly suggest that you make sprouted-grain products a diet staple and use non-sprouted (enriched wheat flour) grains in limited quantities. Sprouted-grain breads, cereals, and pasta can be found at your local health food store.

Legumes

Legumes are a type of plant that contain edible seeds inside their pods, such as aduki beans, black beans, black-eyed peas, chickpeas (garbanzo beans), great northern beans, green beans and peas, kidney beans, lentils, lima beans, pinto beans, and soybeans. Peanuts are also considered legumes because they grow underground, but unlike beans and peas, they form a tuberous growth on the root of the plant. Legumes are packed with nutritional value, providing a balance of proteins and complex carbohydrates, and are typically low in calories as well.

However, legumes—with the exception of lentils—can create acidic conditions in the body, especially peanuts and peanut products, chickpeas, green peas, and most beans. When these foods are digested and metabolized, they leave behind a residue of uric acid that contributes to acidosis. Still, feel free to eat them in moderation because of their nutritional benefits. You should also consider sprouting legumes, a process that involves storing them in a sealed container with water, and rinsing and drying them twice a day until they finally sprout, which may take only one day or up to five. Sprouted legumes are less acidifying and even richer in nutrients.

Meats, Poultry, and Fish

Due to their high protein content, all meats, meat byproducts, poultry, fish, and animal products like eggs cause body acidification. When such foods are digested and metabolized, they produce uric acid residue, which can accumulate to form toxic acid buildup and lead to chronic acidosis. Animal fats such as butter and bacon grease, commonly used to cook and deep-fry foods, are high in saturated fatty acids that add to acidic pH levels. They are also difficult to properly metabolize, and insufficient digestion of saturated fatty acids results in even more toxic waste products that intensify the acidic burden on the body. Compounding this problem is the presence of acid-forming minerals like phosphorus and sulfur in meat, as well as the hormones, pesticides, steroids, and antibiotics often found in products that come from commercially raised sources. These chemicals, most of which are very acidifying, further upset acid-alkaline balance and are simply not good for you to ingest.

Unfortunately, the standard American diet is one that is high in animal and other saturated fats, and thus very acidifying. It's no wonder that acidosis is quite common among our population, not to mention other diet-related diseases like obesity. Even so, it's not necessary to cut meats and poultry completely out of your diet, as a certain amount of animal protein contributes to balanced nutrition. Furthermore, most types of fish are loaded with omega-3s, essential fatty acids that have been shown to reduce the risk of inflammation and other chronic degenerative diseases. But you should limit your intake and always choose foods that are organic, free-range, or wild-caught.

Milk and Milk Products

Like meat, milk and milk products (or dairy) are good sources of protein, which means they are broken down into acids during the digestive process, in turn affecting pH balance. More specifically, milk and milk-based products contain the mucus-causing protein *casein* as well as lactose, a form of sugar that is converted into lactic acid and often difficult to digest. Adding to milk's acidifying effects is its chemical content, which is typical of commercially produced brands. Hormones, antibiotics, pesticides, and hundreds of other substances used to increase milk production are fed to cows and ultimately end up in our milk and dairy supply. As such, milk and dairy should be consumed in moderation, but you do not have to do away with them. After all, milk products contain plenty of vitamins and minerals like calcium, which support bone health and immunity.

Nuts and Seeds

When consumed, nuts and seeds lower pH levels and promote acidity because of their phosphorous, sulfur, and fat content. The only exceptions to this rule are Brazil nuts and almonds, two nuts that are rich in nutrients and antioxidants. (See page 91.) However, pumpkin seeds, sesame seeds, sunflower seeds, cashews, hazelnuts, pecans, and walnuts can all have acidifying effects when digested. But because nuts and seeds have such high nutritive value, it's a good idea to continue to eat them, just in more moderate amounts. You can also reduce their acidifying effects by soaking them in water overnight and allowing them to sprout.

Processed and Refined Foods

The rates of diabetes, heart disease, and obesity among our population today are rapidly spiraling out of control, and the multitude of processed foods in supermarkets and restaurants is one of main reasons why. Some sources estimate that 90 percent of the money Americans spend on food is for products that are processed and refined—meaning that they have been chemically treated, altered from their natural state, and bagged, boxed, or canned. This includes everything from cookies, doughnuts, and other snack foods to commercial cereals and pasta to the fries and hamburgers served at fast food restaurants.

Eating these foods on a regular basis is detrimental to your health for several reasons, including the fact that they're generally nutritionally empty, stripped of their vitamins and minerals. As you might expect, processed foods are also highly acidifying, since they contain significant amounts of sugar and hydrogenated (or partially hydrogenated) oil, a substance used to prolong shelf life. Along with artificial chemical flavorings, food coloring, and preservatives, these substances act as poisons in the body, disrupting acid-alkaline levels and paving the way for chronic disease. If you want to reduce your risk of serious health problems like cancer, you should completely cut processed and refined foods from your diet.

Soda

The acidifying action of soda is twofold, since it contains high amounts of both sugar and caffeine—two substances that we have already established as unhealthy and acid-forming. Soda is also loaded with chemicals that act as toxins in your body, further adding to acid-alkaline imbalance and other adverse conditions. According to Sang Whang, an ionized water pioneer and author of *Reverse Aging,* you must consume thirty-two glasses of water in order to neutralize a single glass of soda. Just recently it was revealed that soda's caramel coloring is created by combining sugars with ammonia and sulfites at high temperatures. The byproducts of this chemical reaction are 2-methylimidazole and 4-methylimidazole, both of which have been documented as cancer-causing chemicals by the United States government.

It therefore shouldn't be difficult to see why soda should be eliminated from your diet. Water—preferably H_2O that is alkaline and has been ionized—should constitute the vast majority of your fluid intake each day. If you still want to enjoy a carbonated beverage every now and then, replace soda with unflavored seltzer water or club soda, but limit the frequency with which you do so.

Sugar

The so-called standard American diet is abundant with sugar-laden foods, whether white sugar, brown sugar, cane sugar, corn sugar, or date sugar. Fructose, galactose, glucose, maltose, mannitol, and sorbitol are other forms of sugar found in a large percentage of commonly consumed foods and beverages. And this is not to mention the honey, syrup, molasses, and other sugar-rich substances used to flavor and dress food.

Sugar, particularly commercial white sugar, poses serious health risks because of how it functions in the body. White sugar, a main component of foods like candy, cookies, pastries, and jellies, is also refined, which means that it's stripped of vitamins, minerals, and enzymes. This absence complicates the processes of digestion and assimilation because the body must call upon its mineral and vitamin stores in an effort to convert sugar into energy. Thus, the nutrients needed to carry out basic physiological functions—such as neutralizing harmful acids—are depleted, disrupting the body's activities and overall stability.

Additionally, sugar serves as fuel for microorganisms such as cancer cells, allowing them to invade and proliferate throughout the body. Even when these microorganisms are destroyed, their decomposition results in fermentation, a process that promotes internal acidic conditions. Acidity, of course, paves the way for diseases to arise. You'll vastly improve your health if you significantly reduce your intake of added sugars, or better yet, eliminate them altogether. Instead, stick to foods that contain naturally occurring sugars like fruit, but eat them in moderate quantities with the exception of alkalizing fruits like lemons, limes, and avocados.

Yeast Products

Excluding baker's and brewer's yeast, yeast products like baked goods, bread, beer, and wine are all acidifying, as are the processed condiments and seasonings in which yeast is used as an ingredient. Moreover, the acidic conditions produced by yeast supports the growth of *Candida albicans,* the bacterium that causes yeast infection (*candidiasis*) and can spread throughout the body. In other words, the overconsumption of yeast can create an environment in which acidity begets more acidity. People who experience yeast infection usually also suffer from medical conditions such as anxiety and depression, bacterial and fungal infections, gastrointestinal disorders, and respiratory problems, not to mention allergies, mood swings, and sleep abnormalities. Therefore, it's important that you limit your intake of fermented foods and refined carbohydrates, while completely eliminating commercial products that contain added sugars from your diet.

Although these foods and beverages have acidifying effects, you should not cut them out completely unless you are suffering from chronic acidosis or otherwise advised by your health-care provider. Include small amounts of acidifying but nutritious foods in your meals while making sure that the foundation of each meal comes from one of the alkalizing food categories outlined in the next section.

Alkalizing Foods

The foods and beverages discussed on the next few pages are the ones that should constitute more than half of your diet—and approximately 80 percent if you suffer from acidosis. A substance has an alkalizing effect on the body when it contains alkaline minerals. Additionally, alkalizing foods do not produce any acidic residues when digested and metabolized, regardless of the amount consumed at any one sitting. Although colorful—especially green —vegetables are touted as the primary alkalizing food, there are plenty of other food sources that can bring your pH levels into balance, including herbs, sprouts, certain fruits and nuts, and cold-pressed oils.

Condiments (Natural)

Herbs, spices, and salts are not typically regarded as condiments, but they are, and they should be a staple when it comes to meal preparation if they aren't already. Cayenne pepper, cinnamon, garlic, oregano, and sage can make your meals more flavorful without the fat, sugar, and other acidifying additives found in processed condiments. Celtic and sea salt are healthful substitutes for table salt, which also promotes acidic conditions in the body. Natural herbs, spices, and salts contribute to balanced acid-alkaline levels while making your food just as tasty.

Fruits

As noted in the previous section, the naturally occurring sugars present in many fruits can result in body acidification. For this reason, it's advisable to eat such fruits in moderation, particularly if you have high blood sugar or weight control issues. There are, however, exceptions to this rule. Avocados, bananas, grapefruit, lemons, limes, and tomatoes are all fruits that strongly alkalize the body when they are metabolized, despite the fact some—grapefruit, lemons, and limes in particular—are inherently acidic. These three fruits are also very oxygen-rich, which adds to their alkalizing capability. Because of these properties, I recommend adding some freshly squeezed lemon juice (or lime, if you prefer) to alkaline ionized water and drinking at least one glass each day. This way, you'll be enhancing acid-alkaline balance and energizing your body simultaneously, making it an ideal way to begin your morning. To reap the most benefits, wait about a half hour to eat breakfast after drinking the glass of water.

Dried fruits are also worth mentioning. Although their sugar content is quite high, they actually alkalize the body, as the drying process rids fruits of their acidity through oxidation. However, you should buy organic dried fruits in order to maximize their benefits, as commercial brands often use sulfur, an acid-forming chemical, as a preservative. In addition, you should monitor your intake of dried fruits due to their concentration of sugar.

Nuts

You already know that the majority of nuts are acidifying (see page 86), but what about those notable exceptions, Brazil nuts and almonds? Unlike the other members of the nut family, these two types alkalize the body. In addition, Brazil nuts contain the mineral selenium, a powerful antioxidant that has exhibited anticancer properties. (Just be sure to limit your intake of these large nuts to one per day, since too much selenium can cause brittle nails and thinning hair.) Almonds are equally beneficial and can be consumed raw or as a delicious drink in the form of almond milk, an excellent substitute for acidifying cow's milk and soy milk.

Oils, Cold-Pressed

Cold-pressed oils are oils that are extracted from their food sources—generally fruits and seeds—without using heat or chemicals, which is the usual commercial method. These standard methods of oil extraction not only destroy some of their nutrients, but also cause the oils to break down during processing, making them more difficult for your body to digest. In contrast, cold-pressed oils are produced at low temperatures by grinding fruits or seeds, and therefore retain their nutritive value. When cold-pressed oils from sources such as borage, canola, evening primrose, flaxseed, grape seed, and olive oil are consumed, the body is fully alkalized. It's a good idea to cook your meals with canola or olive oil, and use the others for flavoring food that has already been prepared.

Sprouts

I've already mentioned the benefits of sprouting foods that are normally acidifying, such as legumes and grains. Sprouting transforms the foods' nutritional content, increasing the amount of vitamins and minerals and improving the foods' digestibility. Proteins, fats, and starches are converted into amino acids, fatty acids, and vegetable sugars that are far more easily assimilated into the body. Additionally, sprouts are rich in energy and other vital nutrients, as well as enzymes and health-boosting proteins.

Most health food stores and supermarkets now sell sprouted beans, seeds, and grains, but learning how to sprout foods at home will make you less dependent on commercial products. The germination process is simple and requires only water, glass jars, and a cool room temperature. Growing your own sprouted foods guarantees their freshness and a limitless supply. The alkalizing potential of these foods is in your hands and literally in your kitchen.

Vegetables

The basis of every alkalizing meal should be an abundance of fresh colorful vegetables. If you are eating for acid-alkaline balance, your lunch and dinner should consist primarily of vegetables that are green, leafy, or brightly colored, such as asparagus, beets, broccoli, cabbage, carrots, peppers, radishes, red onions, spinach, yellow squash, and zucchini. All of these vegetables—and more—are excellent sources of alkalizing minerals and salts, enzymes, fiber, vitamins, and other phytonutrients. But green vegetables are the most beneficial because they contain *chlorophyll*, a substance that cleanses the body and promotes good health. Ideally, a sizeable portion of the vegetables you eat each day should be raw, and the rest, sautéed or steamed. Cooked foods tend to be less alkalizing, and overcooking vegetables causes the deactivation of certain enzymes needed for healthy digestion.

However, there are a few considerations when it comes to buying and eating your vegetables. Because unrefined food is now widely available in health food stores, supermarket chains, and local farmers' markets, you should opt for organic produce over commercially grown brands. Organic produce is also free of pesticides and other chemicals used to grow and preserve conventionally harvested vegetables, so you can be assured that you are not putting unnecessary toxins in your body. Of course, you should always wash your produce thoroughly before eating, regardless of where you purchase it. Using acidic ionized water will ensure that both bacteria and toxic chemicals are neutralized. Finally, if you have a sugar sensitivity (for example, hypo- or hyperglycemia), you should avoid eating vegetables in which naturally occurring sugars are prominent, such as beets, carrots, and squash. When the problem is stabilized, these foods can be gradually reintroduced to your diet and eaten in moderation.

When consumed together with alkaline ionized water, these foods will allow you to achieve acid-alkaline balance as well as reap all the benefits that come along with it. By creating a daily diet derived from mostly alkalizing sources and minimizing your intake of acidifying foods, you will boost your body's ability to maintain good health.

FOOD COMBINING TIPS

In order to optimize the health benefits of your diet, you should know a thing or two about food combining, which is an important part of nutrition. Proper *food combining* means creating meals and snacks based on the compatibility of certain foods during digestion. For example, foods high in protein like fish, poultry, and meat are digested in the stomach, necessitating a very acidic environment. Conversely, starchy foods rich in carbohydrates like bread, potatoes, and pasta begin to be digested immediately upon being chewed and end the process in the small intestine, which requires mildly alkaline conditions. As you can see, when you eat high-protein and high-carbohydrate foods in combination, two entirely different processes must take place simultaneously in order for digestion to be successful. This simply isn't possible. Instead, the foods—both the meat and the potatoes—remain partially undigested in your body, causing many of their nutrients to go to waste.

Furthermore, the undigested food components build up in your colon, where they decompose and then ferment to produce harmful toxins and mucus.

By pairing the right foods together, however, this common problem can be avoided, thus enabling you to maximize the nutritive value of your meals. Here are some basic guidelines for food combining, which will help you make smarter, healthier food choices that support acid-alkaline balance.

- Don't eat foods high in protein (dairy, fish, meats, poultry) with starchy carbohydrates (potatoes, yams, wheat and grain products). This includes meals like steak and potatoes and popular sandwiches like chicken salad, roast beef, tuna fish, and turkey.

- If you want to include a carbohydrate in a protein-centered meal, choose carbohydrate-rich vegetables that are non-starchy such as leafy greens. Most colorful produce—like cabbage, carrots, and squash—is also part of this category. These vegetables do not interfere with the digestion of either proteins or starchy carbohydrates.

- Fruits work better as snacks than as meal staples, with the exception of avocados and tomatoes.

- Try not to drink water with your meals, especially those meals that include foods rich in protein, as you risk diluting the digestive juices needed to break down solid foods. Instead, consume water twenty minutes before eating or an hour afterwards.

- Chew your food thoroughly before swallowing to aid the digestive process.

Using these guidelines to create your meals and snacks will make it easier for your body to not only digest and absorb the foods you eat, but also reap the most nutritional benefits from them. Proper food combining boosts energy and metabolism naturally, and, by relieving the burdens placed on your body, you will soon notice positive differences in how you feel.

CONCLUSION

As this chapter has shown, acid-alkaline balance is vital to achieving optimal wellness. Everything you eat and drink influences the levels of acidity or alkalinity in your body, so a diet that takes this fact into account is important. A pH-balanced diet is particularly relevant for ionized water drinkers, as overconsumption of acidifying foods can quickly undo the powerful healing effects of alkaline ionized H_2O. In order to truly turn your health around, alkalizing water *and* food are both of paramount importance. Additionally, learning how to properly combine your food will enhance both your digestion and the nutritional value of your meals so that you can literally eat and drink for your health. In combination with regular ionized water intake, a daily diet abundant in green vegetables, sprouted grains and legumes, and other alkalizing foods will put you on the road to greater health, greater energy, and freedom from disease.

8

A Guide to Buying and Using Water Ionizers

After reading the first seven chapters of this book, you have all the information needed to put yourself on the fast track to better health and energy. By now, you understand the central importance of proper hydration and acid-alkaline balance to your well-being, as well as how these two are intimately connected. In addition, you have become familiar with the phenomenon of water ionization to create H_2O identical to that of glacier-fed Hunza water, which has brought optimal health and longevity to the Hunza people for centuries. You have a thorough knowledge of ionized water's healing capability, from its internal functions as an antioxidant and alkalizing agent to its external uses as a powerful disinfectant. And finally, you have been given nutritional guidelines for achieving acid-alkaline balance with your diet so that you can maintain the powerful benefits of ionized water. But there's still one thing missing—a water ionizer.

Like any major purchase, buying a water ionizer is an investment that requires careful consideration and research. Ionizers are not cheap, so it's important that you buy one of good quality that fits your individual health needs as well as budget—and you need the right information to do so. The internet can serve as a valuable resource or it can be a consumer trap, as it offers both a wealth of helpful information and manipulative advertising schemes. Furthermore, because water ionizers are sophisticated machines, you should absolutely understand how they work, how you should use them, and how you should *not*—especially when it comes to matters of health. This chapter, therefore, is meant to be a buyer's and user's guide to water ionizers so that your transition to a healthier lifestyle is easier, safer, and stress-free.

BUYING YOUR WATER IONIZER

While reading this book, you may have checked the price range for a standard water ionizer. If so, you already know that ionizers typically range in price from $1,500 to $2,000 on average, to as much as $5,000. Clearly, it's not a purchase that should be taken lightly. At the same time, price should not be a deterrent. If you're uncertain about whether you can afford an ionizer, consider how much money you spend annually or even monthly on bottled water, which is now a grocery-list staple in most households. If you drink even a single 16-ounce bottle of water per day priced at $1.50, you end up spending more than $500 each year—and that's for only one-fourth of your daily water requirement. The figure becomes astronomical when calculated over a decade or more. Purchasing a water ionizer may require you to pay more than $1,000 upfront, but your water expenses essentially end with the initial transaction.

Still, you want to be sure that the money you lay out is well spent. Like any appliance, water ionizers are only cost-efficient if they are reliable, quality-assured, and manufactured by a company with a good reputation. Purchasing an ionizer that meets your individual needs as well as those of your family is equally—if not more—important. As you research and compare different ionizers, consider the following questions:

- **What is the pH range of the water produced by the ionizer?** Generally speaking, if the ionizer does not produce water with a pH range of at least 4 to 9.5, you should not consider buying it.

- **Is the control panel user-friendly?** While it's important for an ionizer to have many settings and options, too many can make its operation confusing. Ideally, the control panel should be straight-forward and not require a lengthy tutorial.

- **How many electrodes/electrolytic plates does the ionizer have?** As you may recall from Chapter 3, the electrodes (or plates), which are located inside the electrolyzing chamber, have a central role in the ionization process. The unit's number of electrodes is one of the main determining factors of the alkaline water's oxidation-reduction potential (ORP)—the more numerous the electrodes, the stronger the ORP. Ionizers can have as many as seven electrodes, but these models produce water with an extremely high pH, making it unhealthy to drink. In general, three or four electrodes should be sufficient.

- **Are the electrodes coated in platinum?** This detail is more significant than it sounds, since a platinum coating ensures protection from water damage. If the electrodes are merely sprayed with platinum, their titanium base can become corroded and compromise the ionizer's overall performance.

- **What type of filter does the ionizer have?** It's generally recommended that you buy an ionizer with a carbon filter, which needs replacing only every nine to eighteen months. Most ionizers have carbon filters, but there are some that use reverse-osmosis with re-mineralizers—as well as other advanced filtering systems—to remove contaminants like fluoride. However, these may give the water a slightly metallic taste.

- **Does the device have any certifications?** There are a number of organizations and agencies on the local, national, and international levels responsible for testing and certifying products according to set standards. Usually, a product's certifications are listed on the manufacturer's website, but you can also contact the company directly for more information.

- **Are you familiar with the manufacturer?** Although there's no rule that says everything is in a brand name, you should also be wary of buying from a company that you've never heard of before, particularly if you're making an online purchase. Plus, well-established companies may be able to offer you a better warranty, which is always something to look for when buying an expensive item. In addition, larger companies may offer free customer service and sell supplementary parts such as filters, thereby saving you money in the long run.

- **Are there installation options for the ionizer?** Most residential water ionizers are intended for countertop installation, meaning that they attach onto the faucet and sit next to the sink. Other models can be installed under the sink and connect directly to your pipes, which you may prefer for aesthetic reasons or if counter space is limited.

Like anything else, deciding which water ionizer to buy all comes down to a combination of practicality and personal preference. Simply by using good sense and exercising some buyer's caution, you can smartly invest your money in a reliable appliance that produces quality water, both acidic and alkaline.

Keep in mind, however, that "more expensive" doesn't necessarily mean "better." There are plenty of ionizers on the market that are both dependable and reasonably priced. Knowing what to look for and what questions to ask will help you avoid falling for common marketing tactics that aim at emptying your pockets. If you do some research, you are sure to find a water ionizer that is appropriate for your lifestyle and financial means. (See the "Resources" section on page 109 for manufacturers and distributors of ionizers located in the US.) The inset on page 101 provides useful information about the misconceptions and realities of water ionizers—knowledge you should have before making a purchase.

SETTING UP YOUR WATER IONIZER

Once you purchase your water ionizer, the next step is installation. If you are using a standard installation method—placing the ionizer on your countertop or connecting the unit directly to under-sink

Ionized Water: Fact or Fiction?

New technology is often accompanied by a multitude of questions and mis-understandings, and ionized water is no exception. As I've traveled around the world lecturing about its health benefits, I've found that there are a number of commonly held beliefs about ionized water as well as ionizers. Let's examine some of these to determine whether they are "fact" or "fiction."

1. **Ionization is not filtration: Fact.** While ionization and filtration are very different processes, every ionizer uses some kind of filtering system. In fact, filters extend the lifespan of the device, since dirty water can cause the electrodes or electrolytic plates to corrode. Pure water cannot be produced without the help of a filter, so make sure you know what kind an ionizer uses before purchasing it. (See page 99 for more about different types of filters.)

2. **Ionized water is a source of oxygen: Fiction.** This misconception is most likely due to the fact that tiny bubbles can be seen in a glass of ionized water, but this is merely an indication of the water's antioxidant strength. Only fish take in oxygen through the stomach; as human beings, we derive our oxygen supply *solely* from the air we breathe into our lungs. However-er, it's true that drinking alkaline ionized water promotes oxygenation of the body by supporting proper pH balance in the bloodstream. The closer the blood is to proper pH balance, the greater its oxygen-carrying capacity.

3. **Ionizers may not rid water of all contaminants: Fact.** Although ionizers effectively remove the vast majority of water impurities, there are a few chemicals like fluoride that are difficult to eliminate. Still, ionizers filter out as much as 99 percent of toxins depending on the filter the unit uses.

4. **Because ionized water permeates cells so deeply and easily, so will the contaminants it may contain: Fiction.** Fortunately, the small amount of toxins that may remain in the water will *not* make it to your cells. You may recall from Chapter 3 that water passes into the cells by way of water channels known as aquaporins, which act as a plumbing system. The aquaporins make the rapid flow of water into the cells possible and filter the water at the same time, blocking the passage of insoluble materials and impurities. Therefore, you do not have to worry about toxins like fluoride seeping into your cells and tissues.

plumbing—hiring a plumber is probably not necessary. Most ion-izers come with instruction manuals that guide you through the process of hooking it up. However, if your ionizer requires custom installation, or if you are using well water rather than tap, you may want to seek help from a professional.

After installing the ionizer, it's a good idea to make sure that it works properly by testing the pH of the water produced. There are three main factors that affect the alkalinity of ionized water—the amount of electrical charge, the amount of minerals in the water source, and the rate of flow of the water across the electrodes or plates. To determine the water's alkalinity, pH testing strips may be used (see page 23), but a digital pH meter—which is cheap and easy to locate online or in a health store—will probably provide a more accurate reading. You can also test the water for antioxidant prop-erties by pouring it into a clear glass and watching to see if tiny bubbles appear. This indicates that the water has good oxidation-reduction potential.

If both of these tests show that your water's pH is still under 8, try running the water at a lower speed—this increases the water's contact with the electrodes, thereby increasing its pH. Additional-ly, do not be alarmed if the water is initially darker in color, as this is simply a result of the filter being used for the first time. Run the water for twenty to thirty seconds and wait for it to return to its normal clear color. If the ionizer continues to produce water that is dark in color, you should call the manufacturer to determine if your appliance is malfunctioning.

It's important that you thoroughly familiarize yourself with your ionizer and read the instruction manual before you begin to ionize water—especially water intended for consumption. When it comes to matters of your health, a responsible and cautious approach is a must.

USING YOUR WATER IONIZER

While the ideal pH for ionized drinking water is 9 to 9.5, you should begin at a slightly lower pH of 8 to 8.5—usually the lowest alkaline setting on ionizers—to gradually acclimate your body. In addition, do not immediately begin to fulfill your entire daily water requirement with alkaline ionized water. Instead, start by drinking one to three 8-ounce glasses—with a pH of 8 or 8.5—per day, and slowly increase the amount and the level of alkalinity each week. By introducing alkaline ionized water to your body little by little, you allow your system to detoxify at a moderate, steady rate. When toxins are pushed out too quickly (due to the water's superior absorbability), uncomfortable side effects such as nausea and headache may occur. Such symptoms may also arise if you consume water with a pH greater than 10, so stick to a healthy range and be careful not to overdo it—there *can* be too much of a good thing. It won't be long before all the water you consume is ionized.

Keep in mind, however, that the time it takes to reach this point varies from person to person. For instance, older adults should incorporate alkaline ionized water into their daily diets at a slower speed than others, as their bodies have had several decades to grow accustomed to acidic toxins. Similarly, people who suffer from chronic acidosis and other health issues should start at the lowest possible setting and gradually increase their drinking water's pH level as their bodies become less acidified. Very alkaline water is not recommended for everyone. Infants, children, and teenagers, all of whom are still growing, should drink only mildly alkaline water with a pH of 8 to 8.5 in order to allow their bodies to develop a natural line of defense against acidity. Ultimately, the pH of the water you should drink depends on your age and level of overall health. You should speak to your health-care provider to determine a healthy alkaline ionized water regimen.

The most important thing is to always listen to what your body is telling you. Here are some other crucial points to keep in mind as you begin to use your ionizer:

- **Do not take medications with ionized water.** Because of how quickly alkaline ionized water is transported and absorbed by the body, it may speed up your system's assimilation of substances. Therefore, the water may interfere with medications, which are intended to take effect in the body at a specific rate. In addition, the water's antioxidant properties may neutralize certain medications. For these reasons, you should make sure that at least a one-hour window separates your intake of medication and your consumption of ionized water.

- **Do not drink ionized water with or close to mealtimes.** Alkaline water can disrupt digestion by neutralizing the acids needed to break down foods into nutrients and wastes. You should avoid drinking alkaline ionized water at least a half hour before and after meals and snacks. Instead, set your water ionizer to the neutral setting (if this is an option), which allows you to drink water that has been filtered, but not ionized.

- **Do not give your pet very alkaline water.** It's understandable if you want to provide your pet with healthy water, but make sure that it is only mildly alkaline. If your pet is very ill, you should check with your veterinarian before allowing it to drink H_2O with a higher pH. In addition, never use alkaline ionized water to fill a fish tank.

- **For optimal benefits, drink alkaline ionized water within a day after first ionizing it.** Although the water's alkalinity can last several weeks, it is strongest in the first three days after it is ionized. Moreover, the antioxidant properties last for only eighteen to twenty-four hours. Therefore, it's best to drink the water when it's fresh and thus more alkalizing, antioxidizing, and rich in electrons.

- **Ionized water can be stored.** If you don't want to drink or use the water immediately, it can be kept in a glass or stainless steel airtight container in the refrigerator. Do not keep the water in an aluminum container, and do not store it for more than a day if you want it to retain its health-giving properties.

- **Never drink the acidic water.** I have noted this important rule before, but it's worth repeating. Drinking acidic ionized water will disrupt your internal balance and may cause oxidation in the body, which weakens the immune system and thus increases your risk of illness.

- **Don't worry about over-alkalinity.** If you have gently eased your body into regular ionized water consumption, there's no reason to be concerned about *over*-alkalizing your body—you can drink as much as one to two gallons each day without any problems. Our bodies produce acids naturally in the course of its daily activities, including breathing and using energy. As long as you're not drinking a liter or more per hour, alkaline water is always highly beneficial.

You will quickly discover the utility and convenience of your water ionizer. Every member of your family can drink water at a pH that is appropriate for their age, level of acid-alkaline balance, and overall health. The water can also be used when cooking to bring out the natural color, texture, and flavor of your food more strongly. Every meal will be delicious. Additionally, alkaline ionized water has a smooth taste that makes it satisfying to drink, and unlike regular tap or bottled water, it will not result in uncomfortable bloating. So drink up, and enjoy!

CONCLUSION

Ionized water may take some getting used to, as it has a slightly different taste than the acidic, chemical-filled tap water we've grown accustomed to drinking. Yet, it won't be long before you'll wonder how you ever lived *without* a water ionizer. This single item can bring you an abundance of energy and better health—it is truly a life-changing appliance. I encourage you to use the information in this chapter to purchase an ionizer that fits the needs of you and your family members, and to produce healthful water for drinking, cooking, disinfecting, and everything in between.

Conclusion

We live in an age in which health is a growing concern, on both national and personal levels. The cost of health care becomes more burdensome each year, and improving its quality and accessibility remains an ongoing and contentious issue. It seems that every week brings another medical study, diet gimmick, or fitness innovation, and the unending abundance of new information makes it difficult to separate fact from fiction. It also makes the important matter of guarding our health a source of stress and confusion—something it should never be. Although the topic of ionized water is no stranger to hype and misinformation, this book has attempted to make sense of a complicated and controversial subject so that you can make informed decisions when it comes to matters of your health and the health of your loved ones.

As with any new technology, the body of research on ionized water is still evolving. But here's one fact that is indisputable: The water you drink has a significant impact on the state of your health. Water is the source of all life, fueling our bodies and giving them the energy, nutrients, and oxygen required to carry out essential biological activities. Unfortunately, the human body requires more water than it is often supplied; moreover, it requires *healthier* water than the kind that flows out of kitchen faucets and sits bottled on supermarket shelves. The combination of insufficient water intake and unhealthy tap water has resulted in a population of people with health problems stemming largely from chronic dehydration and chronic acidosis—conditions that have yet to be made part of the prevailing medical conversation.

Ionizing water is a way to solve this rising health crisis. By drinking alkaline ionized water regularly, you can return your body to its natural state of internal balance and reverse many chronic conditions, from allergies to cancer. By using acidic ionized water topically, you can ensure that you, your food, and your home are protected from harmful toxins and bacteria that promote disease. Water may be a factor in many health issues, but it can also—and should—be the key to preventing and curing them. Scientific advances have made it possible for each of us to produce water that is as life-giving and health-promoting as Hunza water, the secret to the longevity and wellness of its population. We can—and should— follow the lead of scientists, medical professionals, and the general public of other countries like Japan, Korea, and New Zealand in using ionized water medicinally to improve the quality of our health, as well as practically to improve the quality of our lives.

After reading this book, you understand the importance of hydration, acid-alkaline balance, antioxidants, and an oxygen-rich body. You also now realize how severe and widespread many chronic disorders and illnesses have become among our population, and, perhaps, among the people you know. It's now up to you to use the information contained in these pages to take control of your health and change your life. It begins with healing waters.

Resources

The following companies manufacture and distribute water ionizers in the United States. A brief overview of each company has been
provided along with contact information so that you can find an
ionizer that meets your specific needs. For product comparisons
and customer reviews, you can consult ionizeroasis.com, an online
retailer of water ionizers from a wide variety of manufacturers.

AlkaViva
452 East Silverado Ranch
  Boulevard, Suite #205
Las Vegas, NV 89183
Phone: (800) 811-0511
Website: www.ionizers.org
*AlkaViva is an authorized
distributor of IonWays, the only
importer of Emco Tech ionizers in
North America (see page 111). Emco
Tech, which is located in Japan, was
established in 1970 and has been a
leader in the ionized water industry
ever since, earning them several
international certificates. AlkaViva's
website provides thorough
descriptions of the ionizers they sell,
as well as informative articles that
give overviews of topics such as pH*

*balance, water contamination, and
the science of water ionization.*

**AlkaZone/Better Health Lab,
  Inc.**
71 Veronica Avenue, Suite #2
Somerset, NJ 08873
Phone: (800) 810-1888
Website: www.alkazone.com
*In business for over fifteen years,
Better Health Lab, Inc. specializes
in products designed to promote
pH balance, including dietary
supplements, water filters, and
antioxidant water. The company
also manufactures three ionizers
that have dual installation, a self-
cleaning function, and a wide
selection of pH settings.*

Chanson Water Ionizers USA
23341 Del Lago Drive
Laguna Hills, CA 92653
Phone: (888) 624-2169
Website: www.chansonalkaline
water.com

Founded in 2000, Chanson has become a respected ionizer manufacturer throughout Asia, Europe, and now, the United States, offering a line of devices designed for optimal performance. The company also provides technical support and a lifetime warranty. Visit their website for a full list of products and answers to frequently asked questions.

Enagic USA
4115 Spencer Street
Torrance, CA 90503
Phone: (310) 542-7700
Website: www.enagic.com

Enagic, a pioneer in the ionized water industry, is the developer and manufacturer of Kangen Water generating systems. Established and based in Japan since the 1980s, Enagic now has corporate head-quarters in a number of countries—for example, Australia, Canada, Italy, and Taiwan—as well as US branch offices in New York, Dallas, and Chicago, in addition to their California location. Their website provides full product descriptions and specifications as well as warranty information. Prices may vary by distributor.

EromHealth.com
2160 North Central Road,
Suite #203
Fort Lee, NJ 07024
Phone: (201) 540-9648
Website: www.eromhealth.com

The product line on EromHealth.com consists mainly of organic food products, including raw meals, supplements, juices, soy milk, and herbal teas. However, they also sell their own ionizer, the Erom Zion model, which produces acidic water, four types of alkaline water, and non-ionized purified water. The online store also sells custom replacement filters.

FujiBio/RichWay International, Inc.
1750 Kalakaua Avenue,
#103-3534
Honolulu, HI 96826
Phone: (808) 589-2800
Website: www.richwayusa.com

FujiBio-RichWay develops and manufactures therapeutic appliances such as the Bio-Mat, which uses ion electricity to boost energy and enhance strength. Their water ionizer, the multifunctional Alka-Life 7000sL, is based on ionizers produced in Asia. Visit the company's website to download the product brochure and view diagrams that clearly illustrate how the device works. FujiBio also offers alternate payment plans.

IonWays, LLC

8745 Technology Way, Suite C
Reno, NV 89521
Phone: (775) 324-2400
Website: www.ionways.com

IonWays has partnered with Emco Tech, the international leader of the ionized water industry, to bring top ionizers such as the Athena, Delphi, and Melody models to the North American market. Both the Athena and Delphi come with a DVD that guides you through the process of installing, using, and maintaining your ionizer. On the company's website, you can find concise descriptions of IonWays products, which also include alkaline drops, cleansing supplements, filters, pH test strips, and an installation conversion kit.

KYK USA

2885 Sanford Avenue SW,
  Suite #12468
Grandville, MI 49418
Phone: (855)-4-KYKUSA
Website: www.kykusa.com

Formerly known as IonQuench, KYK is the producer of the G^2 ionizer, an advanced model with several different pH settings. The KYK website provides a comprehensive overview of the ionizer, including control panel options and wellness and safety features. The company also has a line of replacement filters and pre-filters, and offers a seven-year warranty.

LIFE Ionizers/LIFE's Pure Essentials

6352 Corte Del Abeto, Suite H
Carlsbad, CA 92011
Phone: (888) 688-8889
Website: www.lifeionizers.com

Family-owned and operated, LIFE Ionizers—a division of LIFE's Pure Essentials—has been in business for nearly fifteen years and is one of the most widely recognized ionizer manufacturers in the industry. Their product line is expansive, featuring countertop, under-sink, convertible, and commercial ionizers. Their website contains an abundance of helpful information, including answers to frequently asked questions, a glossary of water technology terms, and demonstration videos for installing and maintaining your water ionizer.

NewCell Detox

5420 Arapahoe, Suite E
Boulder, CO 80303
Phone: (888) 624-2221
Website: www.newcelldetox.com

NewCell Detox develops technology aimed at ridding the body of environmental pollutants in order to eliminate health problems. Their products include detoxifying foot baths, laser therapy equipment, and two ionizers with many pH settings. The company also manufactures the Alkaline Water Stick, a portable and compact device that converts regular tap water into ionized water.

Solar-Force Corporation

979 Main Street
Stone Mountain, GA 30083
Phone: (877) 468-1110
Website: www.solarforce.com

Solar-Force, a company committed to renewable energy, is a retailer, distributor, and installer of state-of-the-art solar technology. Their website provides descriptions of their three ionizer models—the Aquarius, Genesis, and Oasis Rejuvenators—as well as general information about solar technology for homes, public organizations and agencies, and businesses. The ionizers are equipped with an automatic self-cleaning function and priced at under $1,000.

Tyent USA, LLC

860 Route 168, Suite #104
Blackwood, NJ 08012
Phone: (855) TYENT-USA
Website: www.tyentusa.com

For over fifteen years, the mission of Tyent USA has been to create cutting-edge health technology. The company has developed three ionizers designed to meet varying wellness needs, all of which are equipped with advanced filtration systems and several pH settings. They also produce and sell the H2Go, a portable pitcher that ionizes, filters, and re-mineralizes tap water so that you can stay healthy on the go. Downloadable user manuals and instructional videos are available on Tyent's website.

Water for Life USA, LLC

Phone: (877) 255-3713
Website: www.waterforlifeusa.com

Water for Life USA is the only US distributor of EOS and Hyunsung water ionizers, models developed in Korea and manufactured throughout Asia. Their products include two countertop units, the Genesis Platinum and Genesis Equus Turbo, an under-sink unit called the Revelation TURBO, and a portable ionizer that connects to both faucets and water lines. In addition, the company sells gently used ionizers at discounted rates, along with customized replacement filters, pre-filters, and cleaning agents.

Watershed Wellness Center

6439 West Saginaw Highway
Lansing, MI 48917
Phone: (888) 826-4448
Website: www.watershed.net

The founder and owner of the Watershed Wellness Center is Bob McCauley, a leading advocate of ionized water. The company focuses on preventative health in the areas of water and nutrition, offering a line of health products that includes raw and whole-food nutraceuticals, air purifiers, saunas, and pure water technology. Countertop and under-sink ionizers, conversion kits, and a transportable water ionizer stick are available through Watershed, which lists ionized water as one of their specialties.

References

Ayebah, B et al. "Enhancing the bactericidal effect of electrolyzed water on Listeria monocytogenes biofilms formed on stainless steel." *J Food Prot* 2005; 68(7):1375–1380.

Bari, ML, et al. "Effectiveness of electrolyzed acidic water in killing Escherichia coli O157:H7, Salmonella enteritidis, and Listeria monocytogenes on the surfaces of tomatoes." *J Food Prot* 2003; 66(11):2010–2016.

Batmanghelidj, F. *Water: For Health, for Healing, for Life.* New York: Warner Books, 2003.

Batmanghelidj, F. *Your Body's Many Cries for Water.* Falls Church, VA: Global Health Solutions, Inc., 1992.

Bialka, KL, et al. "Efficacy of electrolyzed oxidizing water for the microbial safety and quality of eggs." *Poult Sci* 2004; 83(12):2071–2078.

Bosilevac, JM, et al. "Efficacy of ozonated and electrolyzed oxidative waters to decontaminate hides of cattle before slaughter." *J Food Prot* 2005; 68(7):1393–1398.

Convertino, VA, et al. "Adequate fluid replacement helps maintain hydration and promotes the health, safety, and optimal physical performance of individuals participating in regular physical activity." *Med Sci Sports Exercise* 1996; 28(1):i–vii.

Deza, MA, et al. "Inactivation of Escherichia coli O157:H7, Salmonella enteritidis and Listeria monocytogenes on the surface of tomatoes by neutral electrolyzed water." *Lett Appl Microbiol* 2003; 37(6):482–487.

Dong, H, et al. "Corrosion behavior of dental alloys in various types of electrolyzed water." *Dent Mater J* 2003; 22(4):482–493.

Dreifus, C. "A conversation with Peter Agre." *New York Times.* January 26, 2009.

Fabrizio, KA, Cutter, CN. "Application of electrolyzed oxidizing water to reduce Listeria monocytogenes on ready-to-eat meats." *Meat Science* 2005; 71(2):327–333.

Fabrizio, KA, Cutter, CN. "Comparison of electrolyzed oxidizing water with other antimicrobial interventions to reduce pathogens on fresh pork." *Meat Science* 2004; 68(3):463–468.

Fabrizio, KA, Cutter, CN. "Stability of electrolyzed oxidizing water and its efficacy against cell suspensions of Salmonella typhimurium and Listeria monocytogenes." *J Food Prot* 2003; 66(8):1379–1384.

Fabrizio, KA, et al. "Comparison of electrolyzed oxidizing water with various antimicrobial interventions to reduce Salmonella species on poultry." *Poult Sci* 2002; 81(10):1598–1605.

Feig, DI, et al. "Reactive oxygen species in tumorigenesis." *Cancer Res* 1994; 54:1890–1894.

Fujino, Y, et al. "A clinical study of liver abscesses at the Critical Care and Emergency Center of Iwate Medical University." *Nippon Shokakibyo Gakkai Zasshi* 2005; 102(9):1153–1160.

Gao, Z, et al. "Observation on the effect of disinfection to HBsAg by electrolyzed oxidizing water." *Zhonghua Liu Xing Bing Xue Za Zhi* 2001; 22(1): 40–42.

Hanaoka, K, et al. "The mechanism of the enhanced antioxidant effects against superoxide anion radicals of reduced water produced by electrolysis." *Biophys Chem* 2004; 107(1):71–82.

Harada, K, Yasui, K. "Decomposition of ethylene, a flower-senescence hormone, with electrolyzed anode water." *Biosci Biotechnol Biochem* 2003; 67(4):790–796.

Hatto, M, et al. "Bactericidal effect of electrolyzed neutral water on bacteria isolated from infected root canals. 64. The physiological property and function of the electrolyzed-ionized calcium Aquamax on water molecular clusters fractionization." *Artif Organs* 1997; 21(1):43–49.

Hayashi, H, Kawamura, M. "Clinical improvements obtained from the intake of reduced water." Dallas, TX: Eighth Annual International Symposium on Man and His Environment in Health and Disease, 1990.

Hiraguchi, H, et al. "Effect of rinsing alginate impressions using acidic electrolyzed water on dimensional change

and deformation of stone models." *Dent Mater J* 2003; 22(4):494–506.

Horiba, N, et al. "Bactericidal effect of electrolyzed neutral water on bacteria isolated from infected root canals." *Oral Surg Oral Med Oral Pathol Oral Radiol Endod* 1999; 87(1):83–87.

Huang, KC, et al. "Reduced hemodialysis-induced oxidative stress in end-stage renal disease patients by electrolyzed reduced water." *Kidney Int* 2003; 64(2):704–714.

Ichihara, T, et al. "The efficacy of function water (electrolyzed strong acid solution) on open heart surgery; postoperative mediastinitis due to methicillin-resistant Staphylococcus aureus." *Kyobu Geka* 2004; 57(12):1110–1112.

Inoue, Y, et al. "Trial of electrolyzed strong acid aqueous solution lavage in the treatment of peritonitis and intraperitoneal abscess." *Artif Organs* 1997; 21(1):28–31.

Iwasawa, A, Nakamura, Y. "Cytotoxic effect of antiseptics: comparison In vitro. In vivo examination of strong acidic electrolyzed water, povidone-iodine, chlorhexidine and benzalkonium chloride." *Kansenshogaku Zasshi* 2003; 77(5):316–322.

Jhon, MS. *The Water Puzzle and the Hexagonal Key*. Coalville, UT: Uplifting Press, Inc., 2004.

Kim, C, et al. "Efficacy of electrolyzed oxidizing (EO) and chemically modified water on different types of foodborne pathogens." *Int J Food Microbiol* 2000; 61(2–3):199–207.

Kim, C, et al. "Efficacy of electrolyzed oxidizing water in inactivating Salmonella on alfalfa seeds and sprouts." *J Food Prot* 2003; 66(2):208–214.

Kim, C, et al. "Roles of oxidation-reduction potential in electrolyzed oxidizing and chemically modified water for the inactivation of food-related pathogens." *J Food Prot* 2000; 63(1):19–24.

Kim, MJ, et al. "Preservative effect of electrolyzed reduced water on pancreatic beta-cell mass in diabetic db/db mice." *Biol & Pharm Bulletin* 2007; 30(2):234–236.

Kiura, H, et al. "Bactericidal activity of electrolyzed acid water from solution containing sodium chloride at low concentration, in comparison with that at high concentration." *J Microbiol Methods* 2002; 49(3):285–293.

Kohno, S, et al. "Bactericidal effects of acidic electrolyzed water on the dental unit waterline." *Jpn J Infect Dis* 2004; 57(2):52–54.

Koseki, S, et al. "Decontamination of lettuce using acidic electrolyzed water." *J Food Prot* 2001; 64(5):652–658.

Koseki, S, et al. "Decontaminative effect of frozen acidic electrolyzed water on lettuce." *J Food Prot* 2002; 65(2):411–414.

Koseki, S, et al. "Effect of mild heat pretreatment with alkaline electrolyzed water on the efficacy of acidic electrolyzed water against Escherichia coli O157:H7 and Salmonella on lettuce." *Food Microbiology* 2004; 21(5):559–566.

Koseki, S, et al. "Efficacy of acidic electrolyzed water for microbial decontamination of cucumbers and strawberries." *J Food Prot* 2004; 67(6): 1247–1251.

Koseki, S, et al. "Efficacy of acidic electrolyzed water ice for pathogen control on lettuce." *J Food Prot* 2004; 67(11):2544–2549.

Koseki, S, et al. "Influence of inoculation method, spot inoculation site, and inoculation size on the efficacy of acidic electrolyzed water against pathogens on lettuce." *J Food Prot*. 2003; 66(11):2010–2016.

Koseki, S, Itok, K. "Prediction of microbial growth in fresh-cut vegetables treated with acidic electrolyzed water during storage under various temperature conditions." *J Food Prot* 2001; 64(12):1935–1942.

Lee, JH, et al. "Efficacy of electrolyzed acid water in reprocessing patient-used flexible upper endoscopes: Comparison with 2% alkaline glutaraldehyde." *J Gastroenterol Hepatol* 2004; 19(8):897–903.

Lee, MY, et al. "Electrolyzed-reduced water protects against oxidative damage to DNA, RNA, and protein." *Appl Biochem Biotechnol* 2006; 135(2): 133–144.

Liu, C, et al. "Effects of electrolyzed oxidizing water on reducing Listeria monocytogenes contamination on seafood processing surfaces." *Int J Food Microbiol* 2006; 106(3):248–253.

Machado, AP, et al. "Microbiological evaluation of gastroscope decontamination by electrolysed acid water (Clentop WM-1)." *Arq Gastroenterol* 2005; 42(1):60–62.

Miracle Water. Japan: NNN/NHK TV, 1996. [http://www.ionlifeusa.com/ en/miracle-water-documentary]. Transcript.

Morita, C, et al. "Disinfection potential of electrolyzed solutions containing sodium chloride at low concentrations." *J Virol Methods* 2000; 85(1–2): 163–174.

Nagamatsu, Y, et al. "Application of electrolyzed acid water to sterilization of denture base part 1. Examination of sterilization effects on resin plate." *Dent Mater J* 2001; 20(2):148–155.

Nagamatsu, Y, et al. "Durability of bactericidal activity in electrolyzed neutral water by storage." *Dent Mater J* 2002; 21(2):93–104.

Nakae, H, Inaba, H. "Effectiveness of electrolyzed oxidized water irrigation in a burn-wound infection model." *J Trauma* 2000; 49(3):511–514.

Nakajima, N, et al. "Evaluation of disinfective potential of reactivated free chlorine in pooled tap water by electrolysis." *J Microbiol Methods* 2004; 57(2):163–173.

Nelson, D. "Newer technologies for endoscope disinfection: electrolyzed acid water and disposable-component endoscope systems." *Gastrointest Endosc Clin N Am* 2000; 10(2):319–328.

Nelson, D. "Recent advances in epidemiology and prevention of gastrointestinal endoscopy related infections." *Curr Opin Infect Dis* 2005; 18(4):326–330.

Ozer, NP, Demirci, A. "Electrolyzed oxidizing water treatment for decontamination of raw salmon inoculated with Escherichia coli O157:H7 and Listeria monocytogenes Scott A and response surface modeling." *Journal of Food Engineering* 2006; 72(3):234–241.

Park, CM, et al. "Efficacy of electrolyzed water in inactivating Salmonella enteritidis and *Listeria monocytogenes* on shell eggs." *J Food Prot* 2005; 68(5):986–990.

Park, H, et al. "Antimicrobial effect of electrolyzed water for inactivating Campylobacter jejuni during poultry washing." *Int J Food Microbiol* 2002; 72(1–2):77–83.

Park, H, et al. "Effectiveness of electrolyzed water as a sanitizer for treating different surfaces." *J Food Prot* 2002; 65(8):1276–1280.

Park, H, et al. "Effects of chlorine and pH on efficacy of electrolyzed water for inactivating Escherichia coli O157:H7

and Listeria monocytogenes." *Int J Food Microbiol* 2004; 91(1):13–18.

Reid, TM, Loeb, LA. "Mutagenic specificity of oxygen radicals produced by human leukemia cells." *Cancer Res* 1992; 53:1082–1086.

Russell, SM. "The effect of electrolyzed oxidative water applied using electrostatic spraying on pathogenic and indicator bacteria on the surface of eggs." *Poult Sci* 2003; 82(1):158–162.

Sakashita, M, et al. "Antimicrobial effects and efficacy on habitually hand-washing of strong acidic electrolyzed water—a comparative study of alcoholic antiseptics and soap and tap water." *Kansenshogaku Zasshi* 2002; 76(5):373–377.

Sharma, RR, Demirci, A. "Treatment of Escherichia coli O157:H7 inoculated alfalfa seeds and sprouts with electrolyzed oxidizing water." *Int J Food Microbiol* 2003; 86(3):231–237.

Shirahata, S, et al. "Electrolyzed-reduced water scavenges active oxygen species and protects DNA from oxidative damage." *Biochem Biophys Res Commun* 1997; 234(1):269–274.

Stan, SD, Daeschel, MA. "Reduction of Salmonella enterica on alfalfa seeds with acidic electrolyzed oxidizing water and enhanced uptake of acidic electrolyzed oxidizing water into seeds by gas exchange." *J Food Prot* 2003; 66(11):2017–2022.

Stevenson, SM, et al. "Effects of water source, dilution, storage, and bacterial and fecal loads on the efficacy of electrolyzed oxidizing water for the control of Escherichia coli O157:H7." *J Food Prot* 2004; 67(7):1377–1383.

Tanaka, N, et al. "The use of electrolyzed solutions for the cleaning and disinfecting of dialyzers." *Artif Organs* 2000; 24(12):921–928.

Venkitanarayanan, KS, et al. "Efficacy of electrolyzed oxidizing water for inactivating Escherichia coli O157:H7, Salmonella enteritidis, and Listeria monocytogenes." *Appl Environ Microbiol* 1999; 65(9):4276–4279.

Venkitanarayanan, KS, et al. "Inactivation of Escherichia coli O157:H7 and Listeria monocytogenes on plastic kitchen cutting boards by electrolyzed oxidizing water." *J Food Prot* 1999; 62(8):857–860.

Vorobjeva, NV, et al. "The bactericidal effects of electrolyzed oxidizing water on bacterial strains involved in hospital infections." *Artif Organs* 2004; 28(6):590–592.

Whang, Sang. *Reverse Aging: Scientific Health Methods Easier and More Effective than Diet and Exercise.* Englewood Cliffs, NJ: Siloam Enterprises, Inc., 1994.

Wilhelmsen, E. "Effectiveness of electrolyzed acidic water in killing Escherichia coli O157:H7, Salmonella enteritidis, and Listeria monocytogenes on the surfaces of tomatoes." *J Food Prot* 2003; 66(4):542–548.

Xin, H, et al. "Effect of electrolyzed oxidizing water and hydrocolloid occlusive dressings on excised burn-wounds in rats." *Chin J Traumatol* 2003; 6(4):234–237.

Yahagi, N, et al. "Effect of electrolyzed water on wound healing." *Artif Organs* 2000; 24(12):984–987.

Ye, J, et al. "Inhibitory effect of electrolyzed reduced water on tumor angiogenesis." *Biol & Pharm Bulletin* 2008; 31(1):19–26.

About the Author

Ben Johnson, MD, DO, NMD

Dr. Ben Johnson—or Dr. Ben, as he is affectionately known to his friends, colleagues, and patients—is a leader in the field of complementary, integrative, and alternative medicine. Dr. Ben, who has always had a keen interest in water research, has said, "If we can have 70 percent of our bodies made of the healthiest water, all other body functions will be better."

After earning his doctorate in osteopathy from the University of Health Sciences in Kansas City, Dr. Ben went on to become both a medical doctor (MD) as well as a doctor of naturopathic medicine (NMD), and is now licensed to practice medicine in five states. In 1996, he cofounded the Immune Recovery Clinic in Atlanta, Georgia, and served as its director for several years. In October 2004, Dr. Ben resigned in order to work full time promoting *The Healing Codes,* a stress-healing program that he used to cure himself of a life-threatening disease.

Currently, Dr. Ben owns and operates Dr. Ben Johnson Services, LLC, which promotes products for natural health care. He is also the cofounder of Thermography, Limited, LLC, a thermography clinic located in Chattanooga, and devotes much of his time to spreading the word about thermography as a safe and effective alternative to radiation-based diagnostic techniques like mammography. Additionally, Dr. Ben consults regularly with patients and health-care professionals around the world, specializing in complementary oncology.

Along with *Healing Waters*, Dr. Ben is the author of *The Secret of Health: Breast Wisdom* and two other health books in the process of completion. Recently, Dr. Ben was featured in the international bestselling book *The Secret* as well as its companion film of the same name.

In addition to his long medical career, Dr. Ben served in the armed forces during the Vietnam War and was a flight surgeon in the Army Reserve for many years. He was also a Senior Aviation Medical Examiner for the Federal Aviation Agency (FAA) for twelve years.

Dr. Ben continues to reside in northern Georgia, where he was born and raised. He lives in Rossville with his wife, Martha, and their two youngest children. He and Martha have been blessed with seven children and seven grandchildren. Dr. Ben is an active member of Gospel Tabernacle Church in Chickamauga, Georgia. In his spare time, he enjoys bee keeping, horseback riding, hunting, skiing, scuba diving, and traveling.

Index

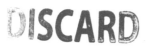